Complementary Alternative Medicine

Should Christians be involved?

Dr Robina Coker

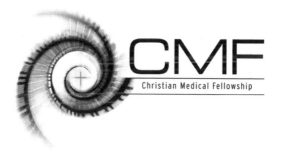

Christian Medical Fellowship

Complementary & Alternative Medicine
Should Christians be involved?

© 2008 by Robina Coker

Published by Christian Medical Fellowship,
6 Marshalsea Road, London, SE1 1HL, England
www.cmf.org.uk

Cover design by S2 Design and Advertising

ISBN 978-0906747384

Body typeset in Palatino 9.5/12

Printed in Great Britain by Stanley L Hunt (printers) Ltd,
Midland Road, Rushden, Northants

Contents

Acknowledgements

My thanks go to Helen Johnson, Julia Sterling, Therese Hoyle, Laura and Nick Hughes, Rosie and Nick Jarvie, Ruth Martin, Bruce McLean, Anthony Metcalfe-Gibson, Rachel Millward and Jeremy Pinkney for their support and encouragement.

I am grateful to my cousin Dorothy Cunningham for her suggestions for source material. Andrew Fergusson provided vision and motivation together with helpful comments. Hilary Gavin made sure I attended weekly gym sessions while writing, thus enabling me to maintain some degree of physical fitness.

Christian Medical Fellowship has over 4,500 British doctors in all branches of the profession as members. It seeks to relate Christianity to the medical world, and medicine to a Christian worldview, and in partnership with others has a growing influence nationally and internationally.

For general enquiries contact:

Christian Medical Fellowship
6 Marshalsea Road
London
SE1 1HL
England

Tel. +44 (0) 207 234 9660
www.cmf.org.uk

CMF and the author regret that they cannot enter into correspondence concerning individual clinical queries.

Introduction

God delights in concealing things; scientists delight in discovering things

Proverbs 25:2
The Message

First this: God created the Heavens and Earth

Genesis 1:1
The Message

If you are reading these pages, the chances are that you have more than a passing interest in complementary and alternative (CAM) therapies. If you are a healthcare practitioner, you are likely to have been asked for your opinion by patients or friends about the value of such treatments. As an interested layperson, you will surely have noted the vast and sometimes bewildering array of CAM products on offer in chemists, health food stores and, increasingly, supermarkets, or know friends or relatives who have sampled therapies such as acupuncture or osteopathy. You may have experienced such treatments yourself. What advice do you give to friends, family or patients about using nutritional supplements, chiropractic medicine, homoeopathy, Bach flower remedies, reflexology, Reiki or hypnotherapy? Do you use CAM therapies yourself? If so, what factors or evidence do you consider before going ahead? This book aims to explore the background to CAM therapies and their relationship with orthodox medicine, and to provide a framework for evaluating the range of treatments on offer.

The inspiration for this book is an earlier title, *Alternative Medicine: Helpful or Harmful?*, co-published by Monarch and the Christian Medical Fellowship (CMF) in 1995.[1] At that time the phenomenon of CAM appeared relatively new, and was seen by many as being inextricably linked to that of the New Age movement. Interest in CAM has since risen exponentially, independently of the New Age.

In 1995 internet access was available to only a few; it now provides information, of variable quality, to hundreds of millions worldwide 24 hours a day, seven days a week. MP3 players, mobile phones and podcasts are transforming the way we obtain news, entertainment and education. Concerns regarding international terrorism fuelled by the attacks in the US on 11 September 2001, dwindling crude oil supplies, and global warming are the subject of daily conversation. Economic growth in China, India, Russia and Brazil challenges the US's long-held position of financial superiority, and the world order established after 1945 is changing rapidly and dramatically. In Western populations obesity and global pandemics of infectious disease are heralded as major public health challenges. These changes affect the priority we accord to our health and how we regard those we expect to preserve and restore healing. The popularity of CAM has persisted and grown, and the CMF considers it is now time to revisit the field. Some of the material in this book is taken from the original; much is new.

Chapter one includes some definitions of CAM. Chapter two puts both CAM and orthodox medicine into a brief historical framework, to enable the reader to understand how medicine is practised in Western societies today. Chapter three examines some of the reasons for the current interest in CAM. Chapter four outlines challenges which may be encountered by patients having recourse to CAM. Chapter five examines how both orthodox and CAM treatments may be evaluated objectively, and how practitioners can be regulated. Chapter six summarises ways in which the reader might use this information. Chapter seven comprises a mini-guide to some of the commoner forms of CAM. The final chapter offers a model for assessment of CAM and provides some illustrative case histories for reflection and discussion.

The CMF is an association of doctors who believe in the truth of the Bible and in Jesus Christ as the Son of God. The opinions expressed in this book are those of the author and do not represent those of all CMF members. Nevertheless, CMF members agree that the Bible is an authoritative source of wisdom in the 21st century, and that orthodox western medicine is a reasonable yardstick with which to compare alternative practices. These principles underlie this book.

Science and the Bible

Approaching CAM from a position of belief in the authority of Scripture is open to criticism in our apparently secular society. Many people assume that science has replaced the Bible. They may therefore argue that the Christian faith is as empirical (that is, knowledge is derived from experience rather than from scientific proof) as the CAM practices under consideration, and should therefore not be used as a reference point. Others may claim that orthodox western medicine has often failed to promote health in our society, and should not be regarded as a yardstick with which to compare other forms of therapy.

Christian faith and scientific reasoning may be held to be incompatible. The Church has in the past sometimes branded scientists as heretics. The most notable example is doubtless that of Galileo, forced by the Inquisition to recant his support of the Copernican system which stated that the earth and the planets rotated round the sun. Others would consider that the whole process of faith (believing without seeing) is irreconcilable with the scientific method, which involves testing hypotheses and accepting only those facts for which there exists objective proof.

There are a number of responses to such criticisms. There exists a wealth of apologetics for the Christian faith derived from objective historical evidence, available for anyone who wishes to study it. The reader could try Nicky Gumbel's *Questions of Life*[2] for a general introduction, or Josh McDowell's *Evidence That Demands A Verdict* for a more detailed study.[3] Evidence for the resurrection of Jesus Christ is presented in JW Wenham's *Easter Enigma*.[4] Christianity is not exclusively based on subjective or personal experience.

The message of the Bible, still the world's number one bestseller, remains wholly relevant for contemporary society. Its unique collection of 66 books, comprising historical and factual narratives, songs and poetry, visions and letters, is neither presented as a mystical account nor as a complex instruction manual for a select few. Instead it invites the reader to participate in the world that God has created and, at the heart of this adventure, to know the Creator himself. Its characters are ordinary people leading ordinary lives, variably thrust into situations of persecution, oppression and exile, war and famine, domestic strife, estrangement, bereavement, despair, hope, reconciliation and celebration. Its moral absolutes, for example the sixth of the Ten Commandments, 'You shall not murder',[5] are valid today and underpin the legal system of Western nations. Among the many themes addressed in its pages are those of trust, truth and justice, and healing, both for individuals and for the communities to which they belong. Trust, honesty, compassion and justice are vital ingredients in healthcare. Healthcare professionals are required to be truthful and honest and show empathy with their patients. Scientists have a responsibility to be truthful in research. Justice in medicine surely means ensuring equal access to healthcare resources for all, regardless of race, gender, sexual orientation, age or financial status. Christians can be confident that the Bible's message remains as relevant for society in the 21st century as in the first.

Although it is clearly impossible to prove or disprove the existence of God using scientific methods, so that their application to this end is unrewarding, mankind has valuable gifts of wisdom and understanding, and these include scientific discoveries. This should come as no surprise if we view science as a means of discovering more about the physical properties of the world that God created. Western medicine is now firmly rooted in scientific principles and research. This does not justify its failings, which reflect instead imperfect understanding and implementation. I consider however that it is quite appropriate to use scientific principles and research at the core of Western medicine to evaluate new therapeutic approaches.

The scope of the book

As in 1995, this book is written with the general reader in mind. I have therefore explained medical terms and principles where they are important to the discussion. I trust this book will help church members to understand the standpoint of much of the medical profession and to clarify their own views. I also hope that some of the ideas expressed here will interest a wider audience. Many in the healthcare professions are concerned by the increased popularity of CAM and wish to preserve the practice of medicine based on established scientific principles and high quality. A more specific readership, of Christian doctors and medical students, is also envisaged.

This book is not an authoritative or exhaustive guide to all forms of CAM practised today. The field is expanding so rapidly that such a guide would be outdated before publication, and in the last few years a wide variety of larger, excellent reference volumes have been published to fill the gap. A few examples are included in the reference section for further reading.[6-8] Furthermore, practices 15 years ago considered unorthodox are now often included in more conventional medical practice. The most notable example is that of osteopathy. The Osteopaths Act, which became law on 1 July 1993, made osteopathy the first branch of CAM to be formally recognised and regulated in the United Kingdom. Another example is acupuncture, now frequently offered by anaesthetists alongside traditional treatment in pain clinics and intensive care units.

Instead I have tried to examine the principles, rather than the specific details, which lie behind both CAM and orthodox medicine, using biblical and scientific perspectives. I hope this will challenge us to look honestly and carefully at any new practice we encounter. Ultimately I expect that more of the truth about CAM will be discovered, and I hope that a scientific and equitable approach to healthcare will be maintained.

To some Christians the topic may seem superfluous. They may view Western societies as gripped by lawlessness, violence and marital breakdown. I alluded earlier to international terrorism, global warming and infectious pandemics. Christians may therefore feel there are more pressing issues to consider than the rights and wrongs of aromatherapy. However, I hope to show that the issues raised by CAM remain important. Some of the questions raised can be applied to other aspects of contemporary life. Finding answers may help us to understand more clearly how we as individuals can influence both the present and the future of the society in which we live.

Increasing interest

There are several further reasons why the CMF considers that CAM merits an up-to-date review. The first is a rapid increase in public demand and clinical practice. Patients and healthcare professionals have shown growing interest in CAM in the last 20 years, in Britain as well as overseas.[9] Surveys in the last decade provide evidence for substantial levels of demand and practice in the UK. In 1998 a postal survey of CAM in England had a 60% response rate from 5,010 randomly selected adults.[10] The results showed that 28.3% had either visited a CAM therapist or purchased an over-the-counter herbal or homoeopathic remedy in the preceding 12 months. Use was lower in older age groups and women were more likely to use CAM than men. The most commonly consulted CAM therapists were osteopaths (4.3% of respondents), chiropractors (3.6%), aromatherapists (3.5%), reflexologists (2.4%) and acupuncturists (1.6%). The authors estimated that expenditure on the principal therapies amounted to £450 million during the preceding year.

In 1999 the British Broadcasting Corporation (BBC) conducted a telephone survey of 1,204 randomly selected British adults.[11] Respondents were asked whether they had used 'alternative or complementary therapies' in the last year, and what specific therapies they had employed. Twenty percent of respondents had used CAM. Most popular were herbal remedies (34% of respondents), followed by aromatherapy (21%), homoeopathy (17%) and acupuncture or acupressure (14%). A smaller proportion had recourse to massage (6%), reflexology (6%), osteopathy (4%) and chiropractic (3%).

In 2000, researchers at the Centre for Complementary Health Studies at Exeter University were commissioned by the Department of Health to conduct a study of CAM in the UK. Their report suggested that there were approximately 50,000 CAM practitioners in the UK and that up to 5 million patients had consulted a CAM practitioner in the previous year.[12]

While presenting evidence to the House of Lords Select Committee on Science & Technology, the Royal Pharmaceutical Society cited a report on over-the-counter sales of CAM preparations drawn up by Mintel Marketing Intelligence in 1999.[13] This showed that retail sales of CAM remedies (herbal preparations, homoeopathic remedies and aromatherapy essential oils) totalled £93 million in 1998. Total revenue had risen 50% from £63 million in 1994.

These figures mirror those from other Western nations. Over one third of North Americans report having used some form of CAM therapy in the previous 12 months, and its use is rising each year.[14] Leading CAM therapies include nutritional supplements and herbal remedies, meditation, chiropractic and massage. Symptoms most commonly treated with CAM include musculoskeletal, respiratory and psychological symptoms. Americans spend at least $50 billion a year on CAM therapies and an increasing proportion is funded by US health insurance schemes.

A similar picture is seen in continental Europe. In 2001 it was estimated that between 20% and 70% of the population have used CAM at some point during their lifetime in those European countries where data are available.[15] In 2005 it was concluded that the most commonly used CAM therapies in Europe are homoeopathy, phytotherapy, anthroposophic medicine, naturopathy, traditional Chinese medicine including acupuncture, osteopathy and chiropractic.[16] The popularity of different therapies does however vary considerably between individual countries.

The phenomenon of CAM has inevitably attracted interest in parliamentary circles. In 1989 the Parliamentary Group for Alternative and Complementary Medicine was established, serving as a political focus for the CAM lobby, and in 2000 the House of

Lords Science & Technology Committee published a comprehensive report on CAM.[13]

Individual doctors now ignore CAM at their own peril and to their patients' detriment. Many of their patients are likely to have recourse to CAM in addition to, or instead of, drugs prescribed by their doctor. Given the possible negative consequences on patients' observance of their doctor's instructions, and the risks of adverse effects, this has implications for all healthcare practitioners. In 2007, a proposal that the UK's National Institute for Clinical Excellence (NICE) should evaluate CAM was debated in the *British Medical Journal*.[17] Professor Edzard Ernst, who holds a chair in CAM at Exeter University, recently stated his view that doctors must give patients evidence on CAM.[18] He points out that CAM appeals to increasing numbers of patients, that patient choice is now an important issue in healthcare, and that much existing information on CAM available to patients is unreliable. He concludes there is an urgent need for doctors to provide accurate patient information on CAM. In recognition of the growing relevance of CAM to mainstream medicine, the Royal College of Physicians, Royal College of General Practitioners and the Prince's Foundation for Integrated Health organised a one day conference in London in September 2007 entitled 'The Science and Art of Healing: Understanding the Therapeutic Response', attended by patient representatives, CAM practitioners and orthodox healthcare practitioners.

The rise in CAM also has implications for medical education. A survey of 117 US medical schools in 1997 reported that 64% offered courses in CAM, either as elective modules or as part of the required curriculum.[19] A 1998 survey in Canada revealed that 81% of 16 Canadian medical schools were including CAM in their curriculum.[20] CAM curricula are being developed within medical schools in the UK.[21] Already some CAM therapies, for example aromatherapy, are being introduced into hospital settings and medical students will increasingly encounter them. Doctors in all fields have a responsibility to teach medical students to apply constructive criticism to the subjects they are taught, and to be ready to challenge new developments if appropriate. The critical study of unorthodox remedies provides an excellent model for teaching medical students the principles of evaluation of any new therapy, conventional or otherwise. It is obviously essential to good medical practice and cost-effectiveness to ensure as far as possible that all remedies offered to the public are safe and effective.

In a broader context, European Union (EU) legislation is currently being applied to CAM. The EU Parliament has adopted several directives regulating the trade of herbal products. Two directives concerning homoeopathy came into force in January 1994, one for human products and one for veterinary products. Directives on traditional herbal medical products and food supplements followed in 2005. Member countries are also reviewing their legislation.[22] Doctors must have a clear idea of which treatments they consider are effective and safe so that they can advise regulatory bodies appropriately and ensure that laws protect patients' interests.

Implications for Christians

Christians believe in one sovereign God, and they believe that he is embodied in the person of Jesus Christ. For them the implications of CAM remedies, some founded on other spiritual beliefs and practices, may cause concern. However, in order to respond wisely it is imperative that Christians are firstly informed of the facts, or they could generate needless fear and prohibitions. Fortunately, considerably more evidence on the effectiveness or otherwise of various CAM treatments is now available than was the case in 1995.

Within the Christian church, the last two decades have brought a revived interest in personal healing, whether physical, psychological or spiritual. Unorthodox remedies may consequently be sampled in addition to more conventional ones, and prayer for healing is not surprisingly regarded by those outside the church as just another form of CAM. While this book does not aim to discuss the issue of 'healing' in the church today, the way Christians approach the subject will have an important bearing on how they view modern medicine. Christian leaders must surely be open to discuss these issues and be ready to apply their biblical knowledge to such situations in a way which will honour God and benefit their congregations.

References

1. Coker R. *Alternative Medicine: Helpful or Harmful?* UK: Monarch/CMF, 1995
2. Gumbel N. *Questions of Life.* UK: Kingsway, 1993
3. McDowell J. *Evidence That Demands A Verdict.* USA: Campus Crusade for Christ Inc, 1972
4. Wenham J. *Easter Enigma.* UK: Paternoster, 1984
5. Exodus 20:13
6. Ernst E (ed). *The Desktop guide to Complementary and Alternative Medicine: an evidence-based approach.* UK: Mosby, 2001
7. Jonas W, Levin J. *Essentials of Complementary and Alternative Medicine.* USA: Lippincott Williams & Wilkins, 1999
8. O'Mathuna D, Larimore W. *Alternative Medicine: The Christian Handbook.* USA: Zondervan, 2001
9. *National policy on traditional medicine and regulation of herbal medicines: Report of a WHO global survey.* Geneva: World Health Organisation, May 2005
10. Thomas K et al. Use and expenditure on complementary medicine in England: a population-based survey. *Complementary Therapies in Medicine* 2001; 9: 2-11
11. Ernst E, White A. The BBC survey of complementary medicine use in the UK. *Complementary Therapies in Medicine* 2000; 8: 32-36
12. Budd S, Mill S. *Professional organisation of complementary and alternative medicine in the United Kingdom 2000: a second report to the Department of Health.* University of Exeter: Centre for Complementary Health Studies, 2000
13. The House of Lords Select Committee on Science & Technology Sixth Report, London UK, 21 November 2000
14. Kamerov D. Wham, bam, thank you CAM. *BMJ* 2007; 335: 647
15. www.cam-cancer.org accessed March 2007
16. *WHO global atlas of traditional, complementary and alternative medicine.* Kobe, Japan: World Health Organisation, the WHO Centre of Health Development, 2005
17. Colquhoun D, Franck L. Should NICE evaluate complementary and alternative medicine? *BMJ* 2007; 334: 507
18. Ernst E. We must give patients the evidence on complementary therapies. *BMJ* 2006; 333: 308
19. Wetzel M et al. Courses involving complementary and alternative medicine at US medical schools. *JAMA* 1998; 280: 784-7
20. Ruedy J et al. Alternative and complementary medicine in Canadian medical schools: a survey. *CMAJ* 1999; 160: 816-7
21. Owen D et al. Can doctors respond to patients' increasing interest in complementary and alternative medicine? *BMJ* 2001; 322:154-7
22. *Legal status of traditional medicine and complementary/alternative medicine: a worldwide review* (document WHO/EDM/TRM/2001.2) Geneva: World Health Organisation, 2001

I

What is CAM?

He is before all things,
and in him all things hold together.   Colossians 1:17

What is health?

In order to understand what lies behind CAM, it is helpful to define first what is meant by health. This is more complex than it might seem initially.

The Collins English Dictionary (21st century edition) defines health as 'the state of being bodily and mentally vigorous and free of disease'. This definition excludes concepts of health in terms of relationships between individuals or of spiritual health.

The World Health Organisation (WHO) goes one step further by defining health as 'a state of complete physical, mental and social well-being and not merely the absence of disease or infirmity'. Although there is no mention of God or spirituality in this definition, the WHO started to acknowledge spiritual issues by 1998, stating that, 'patients and physicians have begun to realise the value of elements such as faith, hope and compassion in the healing process.'[1]

A fuller discussion of possible definitions of health from a Christian viewpoint has been presented by David Atkinson.[2] He starts with Jesus Christ as his reference point in deciding what constitutes a healthy human being. From the creation story recorded in the opening chapters of Genesis, the first book of the Bible, he shows that God intended human life to be lived in a satisfying physical environment in companionship with other human beings, as well as in a fulfilling relationship with himself.

The most casual observer of human life or history will note that this ideal has not been achieved. Christians explain this situation as resulting from the effects of sin. Sin, a most unpopular word in contemporary society, can nevertheless be defined quite simply as any violation of a principle or standard. Christians define sin more specifically as any violation of standards established by God. This includes all rebellion against God. The Bible proclaims that the effects of sin are to shatter the relationship that exists between people and God, and to disrupt people's relationships with each other. Wider evidence of the consequences of sin can be seen in the crime and injustice that corrupt human society and in the devastation of our environment.

One consistent theme running through the Old Testament is the way in which people fail to measure up to God's standards. However, the Bible does not stop there. The New Testament presents God's solution to sin: forgiveness through faith in Jesus Christ. When God forgives sins, he does not ignore them or lightly dismiss human guilt. Instead, God considers the death of Jesus Christ through crucifixion as a sacrifice that pays for the sins of humankind. Those individuals who accept God's offer of forgiveness receive new life, and this gives them the freedom to choose to reject sinful behaviour and to obey God's principles instead.

The word 'salvation' is used in the Bible to symbolise this deliverance of God's people from sinful actions and their consequences. Salvation includes physical, psychological and spiritual healing. Such healing is illustrated by Jesus Christ's works during his life on earth, and described in the factual accounts known as the Gospels. Restoration of relationships between individuals, within communities, and between humanity and the environment, is described later in the New Testament, in a collection of letters written to newly established churches called the Epistles. However, the New Testament also makes it clear that healing in all its fullness is not promised until such time as a new heaven and new earth are established. David Atkinson concludes that the Bible views health as a holistic concept which includes 'individual and social, physical and mental, temporal and spiritual life', and he is clear that wholeness of this kind can only ever be partial in the life we live now.

Some may prefer to ignore a spiritual dimension to health on the basis that it is unscientific to include it. Such readers might consider that there are psychiatrists who will testify to recognising the existence of forces of evil which they had not previously believed in. Some have subsequently reconsidered the possibility of the existence of God. Others have gone further and claimed that a spiritual dimension is essential if modern psychiatry is to understand human nature and behaviour more fully.

An example is Dr Scott Peck. He writes: 'In common with 99% of psychiatrists... I did not think the devil existed. Still, priding myself on being an open-minded scientist, I felt I had to examine the evidence... So I decided to go out and look for a case [of demon possession]. Referrals trickled in. The first two cases turned out to be suffering from standard psychiatric disorders, as I had suspected, and I began making marks on my scientific pistol. The third case turned out to be the real thing... I now know Satan is real. I have met it.'[3]

That health should have a spiritual dimension should not be so surprising, even in the 21st century. After all, science sheds no real light on questions of purpose or morality. No doubt all of us wonder at some stage in our lives why we are here and what our purpose is, or why the world is witness to so much pain and suffering. Answers to 'spiritual' questions such as these are not readily found in scientific study, but rather in the spiritual realm.

What is medicine?

Having attempted to define health, we need to consider definitions of medicine. The Collins English Dictionary (21st century edition) defines medicine as 'any drug or remedy for use in treating, preventing or alleviating the symptoms of disease'. This obviously embraces both medical and surgical interventions. If we accept the holistic definition of health given above, this definition will be seen to be narrow, since it excludes the concepts of social health and spiritual well-being. However, for the present discussion I will use the dictionary definition of medicine as a working basis. I have chosen to do this because it is the concept with which doctors, nurses, physiotherapists and other healthcare professionals are most familiar.

What is CAM?

Even using a fairly narrow definition of medicine, CAM is surprising difficult to define. The title is used to refer to a diverse collection of therapies and disciplines not generally considered to be part of mainstream medical care in Western healthcare systems. Sceptics might suggest that CAM should be defined as all those therapies for which there is no evidence to support their effectiveness. However, while it is clear that some medical and surgical practices have been fully validated by scientific evidence and clinical trials, a large number of apparently well-established and effective orthodox treatments have never been subjected to objective evaluation. It is therefore impractical to define CAM as those therapies not proven to be effective by clinical trials.

Several professional bodies have attempted to define CAM. In 1993 the British Medical Association (BMA) suggested the term 'non-conventional therapies' to describe 'those forms of treatment which are not widely used by the conventional healthcare professions, and the skills of which are not taught as part of the undergraduate curriculum of conventional medical and paramedical healthcare courses'.[4] However, this definition is now unworkable. As noted in the Introduction, many medical schools in the UK and overseas now offer specific optional modules or introductory courses on CAM as part of their core curriculum. Furthermore, use of some CAM therapies is growing among conventionally trained doctors.

Professor Edzard Ernst holds a chair in CAM at Exeter University and has defined CAM as follows: 'Complementary medicine is diagnosis, treatment and/or prevention which complements mainstream medicine by contributing to a common whole, by satisfying a demand not met by orthodoxy or by diversifying the conceptual frameworks of medicine'.[5] However, this definition assumes that all CAM is truly complementary to orthodox medicine, and does not embrace CAM therapies which are offered by their practitioners as alternatives to conventional medicine.

The CAM community itself has failed over the last 20 years to agree on a single definition. In the US, the federal government's lead agency for scientific research on CAM is the National Center for Complementary and Alternative Medicine. This body defines CAM as 'a group of diverse medical and health care systems, practices and products that are not presently considered to be part of conventional medicine.'[6]

A broader, practical definition is provided by the Cochrane Collaboration. The Cochrane Collaboration was founded in 1993 and named after the British epidemiologist, Archie Cochrane. It describes itself as an 'international not-for-profit independent organisation, dedicated to making up-to-date, accurate information about the effects of healthcare readily available world-wide'.[7] It produces and disseminates systematic reviews of healthcare interventions, mainly in the form of the Cochrane Database of Systematic Reviews, published quarterly. These have international standing as well-respected sources of information for healthcare professionals. The Cochrane Collaboration defines CAM as 'a broad domain of healing resources that encompasses all health systems, modalities, and practices and their accompanying theories and beliefs, other than those intrinsic to the politically dominant health systems of a particular society or culture in a given historical period'. This definition is particularly helpful because it allows for variation between different cultures and sets CAM in a historical framework.

Holistic or complementary?

'Holistic' and 'complementary' are other terms frequently used synonymously with 'alternative' medicine. In recent years the term 'complementary and alternative medicine', or CAM, has become popular and gained international acceptance. Nevertheless, I would question whether CAM is necessarily either more holistic, or complementary to, established clinical practice.

The expression 'holistic' merely means that in treating diseases, consideration is given to the complete person. In routine clinical practice this should include an informal assessment of the patient's intelligence and personality; their understanding of, and attitude towards, their illness; and some insight into their financial and social resources. It should also include a thorough assessment of co-existing medical conditions and treatments they are already receiving.

Medical students are introduced to these principles throughout their clinical course and the skills needed to perform such an assessment are gradually acquired during subsequent years. Within the limitations of the busy NHS, such an assessment should therefore be part of good medical practice and not the prerogative of CAM practitioners. Such considerations are in any case vital if the doctor is to decide on the most appropriate treatment and help ensure that the patient is able to receive it.

Furthermore, certain CAM therapies, such as osteopathy, apply a mechanistic rather than holistic approach to disease. This means that, in treating back pain, the primary concern of the osteopath is to restore correct function to the musculoskeletal system, emphasising the role of physical treatment. A good osteopath will enquire about emotional and psychological stresses in the patient's life, which may for example alter the patient's attitude to pain or disability. There is however no implicit reason to suppose that the outlook of the osteopath is any more holistic than that of a caring and competent general practitioner. That the term holistic has come to be synonymous with CAM is to some extent an indictment of orthodox medicine, as we shall see later.

The 'complementary' label implies that orthodox medicine is in itself incomplete. This is undoubtedly true, since there will always remain scientific and therapeutic advances to be made, and doctors being human are regrettably fallible. Christians may in addition consider that orthodox medicine alone cannot treat the soul, perhaps exemplified by the failure of modern antidepressants such as Prozac to rid Western populations of an epidemic of depression. Nevertheless there are several reasons why I consider that CAM is not always complementary to established practice.

Firstly, it has been shown that some substances present in herbal remedies are not harmless but in fact quite toxic. Evidence for this is discussed in chapter four. Since these substances have not been subjected to safety tests, such side-effects are in many cases unpredictable and may thus in some circumstances be extremely dangerous. I therefore think it is only prudent to restrict the use of the word 'complementary' to those therapies that have been formally evaluated, both for efficacy and safety, along the lines described above.

Secondly, some therapies such as homoeopathy are based on principles that conflict fundamentally with the principles underlying orthodox medicine. The basic mechanisms by which orthodox pharmaceutical agents exert their effects are generally known, at least in outline. A drug has to interact with a molecule (usually a protein) in the body before it can produce a therapeutic effect. It may bind to a specific receptor (a molecule, typically on a cell membrane, which 'recognises' the drug) or it may interact with a biological catalyst (an enzyme) responsible for controlling a biochemical reaction in a cell. This interaction leads to an alteration in cellular function. If the cell belongs to the organism, and if sufficient drug molecules are present, this will lead to altered tissue function and subsequently to changes in organ function.

Alternatively, if the cell targeted by the drug is a foreign one, such as a bacterial cell, bacterial function will be altered and the bacterium will ultimately die. Owing to the way drugs act, their pharmacological effects are related to their concentration at the site of action. Within certain limits, the higher the concentration, the greater is the resulting pharmacological effect. This 'dose-response relationship' is well established for drugs currently on the market, and is the basis of normal prescribing practice.

The practice of homoeopathy is based on entirely different principles. The active ingredient in homoeopathic remedies is diluted in an inactive vehicle such as water or alcohol until no molecule of the original active compound remains. According to the rational approach described above there is no reason to suppose that the active ingredient can be effective, since it is no longer physically present. However, homoeopathic practitioners believe that by subjecting this solution, now consisting only of the vehicle, to a series of shakes, called succussions, it becomes more potent. These claims run completely contrary to the principles underlying modern drug therapy. It is therefore not possible to reconcile them in the light of our present understanding or to consider homoeopathy as being complementary to orthodox medicine.

It has been argued that since CAM practitioners are not capable of making a careful diagnosis, they should always work alongside orthodox medical practitioners who will make the diagnosis and then refer for treatment.[8] The term 'alternative' is thought to be ill-conceived and 'complementary' more appropriate. However, I believe that this underestimates the quite competent evaluation that, for example, an osteopath can reach after a careful history and clinical examination.

The expression 'alternative' in my view accurately summarises the standing of many CAM therapies at present. In some cases they may become complementary to orthodox medicine, but only after rigorous evaluation.

What is the 'New Age'?

A full discussion of the New Age is outside the scope of this book. However, the Collins English Dictionary (21st century edition) defines New Age as a 'philosophy characterised by a belief in alternative medicine, astrology, spiritualism, etc'. No discussion of CAM is thus complete without reference to the New Age.

The contemporary term 'New Age' is used in a Western context where the Judeo-Christian tradition remains predominant in spiritual circles, and many New Age ideas and practices contain criticisms of organised mainstream Christianity. The currently used phrase 'New Age' was coined by Annie Besant at the beginning of the 20th century. She later became the leader of the Theosophical Society. Founded in 1875, the society embraced beliefs derived from the sacred writings of Brahmanism and Buddhism. The expression 'New Age' is derived from the astrological theory that each 'star-age' lasts for 2,000 years. Adherents of the New Age philosophy claim that we have left the age of Pisces, the fish, a sign identified with Christianity, and are entering the age of Aquarius, identified with humanism.

Key tenets of this philosophy include pantheism – all that exists is god, and so, by implication, we are all gods, and relative rather than absolute morality – good and evil are only illusions, therefore each individual must decide his or her own morality. Rather than follow the lead of organised religion, New Agers typically construct their own spiritual journey from a mixture of mystical traditions from other religions, including shamanism, neo-paganism and occultism. Contemporary proponents of the New Age movement include Shirley MacLaine, whose 1987 television mini-series *Out on a Limb* was an autobiographical account of her mid-life spiritual exploration, Helen Schucman, Jane Roberts, James Redfield, Marlo Morgan, Neale Donald Walsch and Glenda Green.

Important New Age themes, though not subscribed to by all followers, include the belief that all life is spiritually interconnected and participates in the same energy; belief in the value of spiritual beings (for example angels) to act as personal guides; belief in reincarnation; an emphasis on renaissance of feminine forms of spirituality; the worth of meditation, yoga and other Eastern practices; the merit of eating locally produced, seasonal organic food to benefit both mind and body; the value of fasting to promote higher levels of consciousness; the use of rocks and crystals to aid healing through their psychic energies; and the conviction that a positive attitude supported by affirmation will achieve success in any desired goal.

Some of the above themes do not immediately conflict with the views of individual Christians, who may rightly fast, meditate and pay attention to a healthy diet. Nevertheless, a clear contrast with Christianity is evident. As outlined earlier, Christians believe that there is one God who is distinct from the world he created and that man is separated from God by sin. Sin may be an unpopular concept today, but everyone recognises selfish anger, lust, envy, hatred and arrogant pride. These are some of the sins condemned in the Bible. Reconciliation with God can only come through faith in Jesus Christ, who said of himself, 'I am the way and the truth and the life. No-one comes to the Father except through me'.[9] God has given his people fundamental principles for living. These are outlined in the Old Testament, in the text we now know as the Ten Commandments.[10] Much later they were summarised by Jesus as 'Love the Lord your God with all your heart, and with all your soul and with all your mind', and 'Love your neighbour as yourself'.[11]

Not all CAM therapies are linked to the New Age movement, but the quest for self-perfection and ever increasing health follows naturally from this philosophy. New Age thinking incorporates astrology, magic and crystal-gazing, and the belief that healing forces are harnessed through crystals and pyramids. A number of CAM therapies do have their roots in New Age thinking. It is because of such considerations that Christians oppose the New Age movement and many are critical of CAM.

However, I believe it is unwise to dismiss all such treatments too hastily. The truth must be sought in each case. It is also important to realise that the so-called New Age philosophy is in fact anything but new: pantheism, astrology and rejection of the concept of absolute morality can be traced back to antiquity, and the term New Age has in fact appeared throughout history to signify a new beginning, whether desired or real. The Christian faith has survived 2,000 years of heresies and persecutions. Christians need to remember this when considering CAM. We can be confident in our God and we are invited to ask him for wisdom when ours seems lacking.[12]

References

1. World Health Organisation. *WHOQOL and spirituality, religiousness and personal beliefs: report on WHO consultation.* Geneva: WHO, 1998
2. Atkinson D. *Towards A Theology of Health* in *Health: The strength to be human.* UK: IVP/CMF, 1993
3. Scott Peck M. *People of the Lie.* UK: Arrow, 1983
4. British Medical Association. *Complementary Medicine: New Approaches to Good Practice.* UK: Oxford University Press, 1993
5. Ernst E *et al.* Complementary Medicine - A Definition (letter). *British Journal of General Practice* 1995; 5: 506
6. www.nccam.nih.gov accessed November 2007
7. www.cochrane.co.uk accessed April 2007
8. Livesey R. *More Understanding Alternative Medicine.* UK: New Wine Press, 1988
9. John 14:6
10. Exodus 20:1-17; Deuteronomy 5:6-21
11. Matthew 22:37-40
12. James 1:5

For reflection on your own or for discussion in a small group

1. How would you define health in a Western society?
2. Would your definition be different if you lived in a developing country? If so, why?
3. How would you define CAM?
4. Do you think CAM is complementary to orthodox medicine, or alternative, or neither? Why?
5. What do you understand by the New Age? Can you see positive aspects in New Age beliefs? How should Christians respond to these?

2

A historical perspective

Whatever is has already been,
And what will be has been before.   Ecclesiastes 3:15

All professions are conspiracies against the laity.   George Bernard Shaw

Why history?
In chapter one a definition of CAM was proposed describing CAM as a 'broad domain of healing resources that encompasses all health systems, modalities, and practices and their accompanying theories and beliefs, other than those intrinsic to the politically dominant health systems of a particular society or culture in a given historical period'. From this it follows that CAM exists outside the context of orthodox medicine, and cannot be considered in isolation from orthodox medicine.

In our search for the background to CAM we therefore need to explore the historical background to orthodox medicine. This will allow us to understand the origins of both orthodox medicine and CAM and put them in perspective. The following historical sketch is of necessity a condensed outline; for detailed accounts the interested reader may want to consult the sources[1-6] at the end of this chapter.

The origins of disease
Our earliest ancestors were nomadic hunters and gatherers, living in scattered groups of around 50 to 100 individuals. Their lifestyle, which excluded domesticated animals, kept the risk of contagious diseases low. The threat of disease came from wild animals which could transmit infections (zoonoses) such as sleeping sickness, tetanus, leptospirosis and yellow fever; parasites such as worms and

lice; and the bacteria present in humans themselves, such as *Salmonella* and *Treponema* (the latter causing yaws and syphilis).

The advent of settled farming communities was one of the most important transitions in the history of humankind. Wild grasses were tamed to become domesticated varieties of wheat, rye, barley and rice. Dogs were probably domesticated first, followed later by cattle, sheep, goats, pigs, horses and poultry. With domestic animals came many new diseases, including parasites. Permanent settlements attracted mice and rats, which often helped to spread disease, together with mosquitoes and other blood-sucking insects.

Agricultural surpluses fuelled the growth of cities, which in turn brought about the spread of infectious diseases. Wars led to epidemics; in some cases armies were wiped out as they encountered previously unknown infectious agents to which they had no immunity. Epidemics of plague recurred throughout Europe from the 14th to the 18th centuries. With the arrival of Columbus in the Americas in 1492, Western diseases such as smallpox, diphtheria, plague, scarlet fever and leprosy spread throughout the continent. It is thought they ultimately claimed the lives of around 90% of the indigenous non-immune populations.

Nutritional diseases emerged. Early hunter-gatherers consumed a very wide variety of foodstuffs. Their descendants, engaged in settled agricultural communities, had however an increasingly limited diet centred on a staple crop. Pellagra due to niacin (nicotinic acid, vitamin B_3) deficiency became widespread in communities depending on maize cultivation for survival. Beriberi resulting from lack of thiamine (vitamin B_1) was prevalent in populations cultivating rice. Scurvy caused by vitamin C deficiency afflicted seafarers, armies, Arctic and Antarctic explorers, and the Irish during the potato famine of 1846, when the substitute grains imported did not contain vitamin C.

Further modern diseases arose as a consequence of industrialisation. Coal workers' pneumoconiosis (black lung disease) caused premature death in coal miners, lead exposure caused poisoning, and working with asbestos led to the lung disease asbestosis. Soot caused scrotal cancer in boys employed as chimney sweeps, the first occupation identified as linked with cancer. In the 20th century there was apparently a substantial rise in the incidence of cancer, heart disease and Alzheimer dementia. Although in part related to increased survival, it is likely that other factors including tobacco and alcohol use and environmental pollutants are also responsible. Greater longevity has led to increased frequency of genetic diseases, since more carriers now survive to pass on the defect to their offspring.

The origins of medicine

All primitive cultures regard religion, magic and medical treatment as inseparable. Religion and magic had a similar aim: the defence of the individual against evil forces. Thus medicine has many origins in magical and religious practices. Primitive dances were frequently part of complex rites invoking the aid of supernatural forces, and early healers sought supernatural origins for most events including sickness. Sorcerers typically formed an exclusive caste to safeguard secrets and heighten their authority. Consequently they usually occupied a high place socially and politically.

Magical medicine thus developed from largely empirical practices. Some practices worked because they depended on the power of suggestion, or what we now term the placebo effect (described more fully in chapter three). Examples include spells and amulets, the latter worn to keep illness and evil spirits at bay. Some practices, however, were based on studying the healing properties of plants and the toxicity of animal poisons. The origin of pharmacology, the science of drugs, lies in the particular knowledge held by all major populations about locally available therapeutic and narcotic (sleep-inducing) agents. Snake venom antidotes were initially derived from such studies. Archaeological excavations of sites thousands of years old provide evidence for other forms of skilled medical attention: broken bones repaired, dislocations replaced and wounds successfully tended.

The origin of medicine is often traced to the ancient Greeks, but they were not alone in their achievements. Ancient Mesopotamia and Egypt had medical texts and traditions predating those of the Greeks, while those of India, China and the Far East have equal claim to antiquity.

The Assyrio-Babylonians believed that disease was caused by demons, and astrology was central to their medical practice. It was held that only doctor-priests could interpret demonic actions and invoke help from the gods. Answerable to the gods, these early medical practitioners nevertheless used many drugs derived from plants and animals, and recognised various fevers, plagues, rheumatism, venereal diseases and tuberculosis. Babylonian texts dated around 650 BC describe epilepsy. Much practice apparently combined ritual and commonsense. For instance, a drink of beer and sliced onion was prescribed for eye trouble. Using onion is logical since it induces the flow of tears which contain lysozyme, an antibacterial agent. Assyrio-Babylonian doctor-priests were highly regarded and often summoned to provide medical services as far away as Egypt. Assyrio-Babylonian surgeons were by 1900 BC developing professional status and answerable to civil authorities. King Hammurabi, king of Babylonia from around 1948 to 1905 BC, promulgated one of the earliest known statutes of law, the code of King Hammurabi. This established scales of fees, and penalties for incompetence and negligence by surgeons.

The Egyptians apparently had a relatively sophisticated national health service. The sick were treated free of charge in wartime and while travelling, and doctors were paid by the state. At the national level there was an emphasis on domestic hygiene, diet, sexual relations and burial. Heart complaints, including angina, and abdominal and eye disorders were recognised, as were various swellings. In about 420 BC Herodotus wrote: '... each physician applies himself to one disease and not more. All places abound in physicians; some are for the eyes, others for the head, others for the teeth, others for the intestines and others for internal disorders'.[7]

India, China and Japan

In the highly structured society of India, doctors likewise occupied a clear niche. The Vedas (*veda* is Sanskrit for knowledge) are a compilation of Hindu texts dating from around 1000 BC containing much medical as well as religious instruction. An empirical and rational system, Ayurvedic medicine (*ayus* is Sanskrit for longevity), replaced earlier magical and religious practices between 600 and 100 BC. Prevention of disease was important, and Brahmin regulations laid emphasis on personal hygiene and sanitation. Surgery was especially advanced and rhinoplasty (reshaping of the nose) was frequently performed to repair noses cut off as punishment for adultery. In the 1950s the Indian plant *Rauwolfia serpentina* (snake-root) was introduced into Europe and its active constituent reserpine used to treat high blood pressure; it was later superseded by other drugs with fewer side-effects. Ayurvedic medicine continues to be widely practised in modern India with state support, often alongside Western medicine, and remains holistic in its approach.

Chinese medicine can be traced back to writings more than 2,000 years ago, and is partly understood in the context of religious beliefs.

In the Taoist legend of the creation of the world, chaos was overcome under the inspiration of the god Pan Ku and order established on the basis of two opposite poles, yang and yin. Yang represents the positive, active, masculine: left-handed, light, sky, dryness and warmth. Yin represents the negative, passive, feminine: right-handed, earth, moisture and cold. Illness was believed to result from an imbalance between these two poles. The emperors influenced the development of medicine and initiated the most typically Chinese practice, that of acupuncture. Herbal remedies were also widely used, including opium as a narcotic, rhubarb as a laxative, and ephedrine (derived from the Chinese herb *ephedra*) for asthma. Iron was given to treat anaemia, kaolin for diarrhoea, and the first attempts were made to immunise against smallpox.

By contrast, little is known of early Japanese medicine. In the 4th century Chinese civilisation penetrated Japan and for many centuries its medicine supplanted native remedies. The Portuguese landing in 1542 introduced European medical practices which were adopted as avidly as the Chinese ones before them.

Hebrew, Greek, Roman and Arab culture

The biblical Hebrew people apparently inherited a number of beliefs from ancient Mesopotamian culture, among them the conviction that disease was divine punishment for sin. However, in contrast to Egypt and Mesopotamia, the monotheistic Hebrews viewed God as their true healer. Belief in one god excluded use of magical practices; resorting to divination, omens, exorcists or sorcerers was forbidden by law.[8] The belief that disease was the outcome of sin was later passed on to Christian medieval Europe. Although the Bible teaches that some diseases can result from sin, there are also instances where it makes clear that disease and suffering occur for other reasons, some not fully explained. The story of Job in the Old Testament and Jesus' own teaching provide examples. [9-10]

Greek medicine is unique in the ancient world because it developed alongside a philosophy disciplined by strict criticism. Healing became a science as well as an art. Magic was gradually replaced by enquiry, and medicine came to be regarded as a science. Attempts emerged to give all phenomena natural rather than supernatural explanations, and medicine in Greece acquired professional status. Schools of medicine were established and pupils had to apply for a licence to practise, only granted when the standing of the school they attended had been considered.

Practitioners were allowed to open surgeries and treat patients for fees. Army and gymnasium doctors (the latter comparable to today's sports physicians) were also licensed. The medical school which was to become the most famous was on the island of Kos, and its most renowned practitioner was Hippocrates (born on Kos around 460 BC). By then physicians no longer regarded illness as the gods' punishment but instead sought rational methods of treatment. Hippocrates was at the forefront of medical science in his time and attempted to classify knowledge under the headings of anatomy, physiology, general pathology, diagnosis, therapy, prognosis, surgery, obstetrics and gynaecology, mental illness and ethics.

Greek culture extended to Asia Minor, Italy and Sicily, and Greek practitioners after Hippocrates gradually infiltrated Rome. The early Roman view was that medicine was supernatural and magical, its practice only appropriate for slaves. Extension of Greek culture gradually changed this attitude, and the Romans later built hospitals for domestic slaves and soldiers in permanent forts in conquered territory.

From 313 AD Christianity was recognised as an official religion of the Roman Empire. The church generally viewed medicine positively and increasingly became the preserver of Western learning. Jews and Christians built hostels for pilgrims; many had some facility for medical assistance even if limited to food, warmth and shelter. In the chaos of wars and plagues troubling Europe in the Middle Ages, welfare of the sick was taken over by religious orders. Monasteries thus provided much of the available medical care, which was therefore controlled by the church. Infirmaries were built in the monasteries and medicines were made from plants cultivated in the grounds.

In the Arab world, Greco-Roman knowledge was translated and preserved. Notable was a Christian Arab, Hunain ibn Ishaq, a 9th century medical scholar in Baghdad. He searched out and translated Galen's work into Arabic and wrote a major tract on eye diseases. The Arabic peoples (including dispersed Christians, Persians and Jews as well as Muslims) established pharmacy and chemistry as sciences, built hospitals and developed knowledge of diseases such as tuberculosis. Training institutions for physicians flourished and in the 10th century the caliph of Baghdad required that all practitioners take an examination before being licensed.

Europe

Orthodox European medical education was later developed in the newly established universities. The most renowned school of medicine was established in Salerno in Italy in the 10th century and reached its height of fame in the late 11th century. Founded on Greek, Latin and Islamic civilisations in the ninth century, it was free of clerical control and open to female practitioners. In 1240 Frederick II granted it the right to license doctors to practise. Permission was given after a five year course of study and one year of practice under expert supervision, a remarkably similar system to that in this country today. The influence of the Salerno school later spread throughout Italy and southern France.

In Northern Europe however, society remained isolated and rural, based on a local agricultural economy. Physicians were available only to the higher ranks of society and the masses relied on folk healers. It is in this context that orthodox medicine arose in Britain. Three types of medicine, or healing, have been described in Britain in the 16th century, when orthodox medicine was beginning to emerge as a profession.[11] The first was *official* (or orthodox) healing. This was endorsed by the newly established medical profession, taught in the universities, based upon physical knowledge available at that time and open to intellectual debate. The second was *practical* healing, founded on folklore and involving the use of herbs and minerals. Contemporary examples of practical healing might include the use of vitamins, arnica, cough remedies and herbal teas. The third was *ritual* healing, consisting of the use of charms, frequently derived from the prayers of the pre-Reformed church, witchcraft and sorcery.

Orthodox medicine was not always superior to the practical wisdom of the day. A striking illustration comes from the outbreaks of syphilis which struck European ports in the late 15th century. Doctors of the prestigious University of Ferrara deemed that the outbreaks resulted from a particular astrological event, while the Aberdeen Town Council pronounced that it was due to the arrival in town of sexually promiscuous women.

From early on the Church was hostile to lay practitioner healing because of its presumed association with magic and witchcraft. Misgivings about female practitioners were prevalent in the 16th century Church and lent further force to the opposition, both witches and midwives being open to attack. The first legal restriction of medical practice came in 1512 when an Act was passed requiring the Church to supervise the competence of physicians. Six years later, concerned both to limit the unofficial practice of medicine and to establish national standards for orthodox medical practitioners, King Henry VIII founded the Royal College of Physicians in London. Orthodox medicine thus eventually emerged as having both political power and a monopoly over the explanation of disease and healing.

During the 15th and 16th centuries, expeditions to the American continents led to international exchange of medical information. Quinine, a drug extracted from *cinchona* bark, was imported to Europe by explorers returning from Peru, where natives had for years used it to treat malaria. This paved the way for introduction of other pharmacologically active compounds. New drugs were gradually proposed, tried and accepted. Medical practice slowly changed from being a mixture of folklore and witchcraft to become a scientific discipline.

Medical progress in 16th century Britain was just as influenced by European scientists outside the medical establishment as it is today. Politicians, engineers, physicists and chemists all contributed. Galileo developed a watch to measure pulse rate, while a contemporary, Sanctorius, designed and built the first weighing machine and clinical thermometer. The microscope had a considerable impact on medical progress in the 17th century. Robert Hooke, in London, was the first to use it to describe cells. This led to a new medical philosophy, expounded by those such as René Descartes, who regarded the human body as a complex piece of machinery. Such an approach may have shocked the religious establishment but it enabled rapid advances in medical science. The study of physiology began in earnest. William Harvey, the first scientist to prove that blood is pumped around the body in a closed circulatory system, is the best known British physiologist of this era.

One British 17th century physician who helped prepare the medical profession for new information provided by medical scientists was the puritan Thomas Sydenham (1624-1689). Basing his practice on that of Hippocrates, he made detailed observations of signs and symptoms. Sometimes refusing to use complex but ineffective remedies, he had a commonsense approach to therapy, prescribing iron for anaemia, quinine for malaria and opium for pain. His work helped establish within the British medical profession a tradition of clinical observation and professional criticism. As a result of this, and because of his concern for medical ethics, he became known as the 'English Hippocrates'.

The Industrial Revolution

In the 18th century, the Industrial Revolution dramatically altered living standards and disease patterns. Huge new factories and towns led to widespread overcrowding and pollution. New housing estates had no clean water, sewage facilities, or space for recreation. One immediate result was an increase in diseases related to manufacturing processes. Several physicians observed the new working conditions and made recommendations, such as masks for miners, and ventilation for workshops. Industrial medicine became a new discipline, although most recommendations were dismissed as too expensive.

The 18th century also saw breakthroughs. Edward Jenner, a clergyman's son from Gloucestershire, revived the idea of smallpox vaccination. Twenty years before, a Dorset farmer, Benjamin Jesty, had vaccinated his wife and two sons with cowpox to protect them against smallpox, having noted that dairymaids who developed cowpox did not get smallpox. The experiment was ignored by the medical profession. Edward Jenner repeated it successfully, and the news spread around the world. During the next 200 years, vaccination, first against smallpox and then against other diseases, was to provide the most effective weapon available to doctors for controlling infectious diseases. James Lind conducted the first serious clinical trial of the treatment of scurvy in 1747, thereby discovering the prevention and remedy in citrus fruit.

The birth of the pharmaceutical industry was at least partly inspired by William Brockenden, from Devon, who discovered that pills could be produced by reliable tablet-making machines, rather than being hand-rolled. This meant that drug doses could be standardised, and pharmaceutical manufacturers could easily boost profit by increasing output.

Early 19th century clinicians applied theoretical knowledge gained by medical scientists. René Laennec in France developed the stethoscope. A long-established practice of selling corpses for dissection climaxed in scandal, and a British Anatomy Act ruled in 1832 that unclaimed dead bodies should go to medical schools for dissection. The study of anatomy was thus affirmed and linked with clinical science.

The Industrial Revolution increased the number of those who could afford professional medical care, leading to greater demand for properly recognised physicians and surgeons, rather than unqualified quacks. Licensing and registration of physicians, surgeons and apothecaries became official. Tuberculosis and cholera raged unchecked in cities; in London the 1848-9 cholera outbreak killed nearly 15,000. Edwin Chadwick, a civil servant, lawyer and journalist, studied the epidemiology of infectious diseases, using maps to pinpoint the worst death rates. He argued that proper sanitation would improve quality of life and be cost-effective. His recommendations were incorporated into a Public Health Act in 1848 and drove the development of clean water supplies and sewage disposal facilities.

Surgical mortality in the 19th century, despite anaesthesia, was 40 to 60%. Patients died from post-operative infections regardless of successful surgery, because surgeons did not adopt precautions against infection. Louis Pasteur, a French chemist, developed the theory that fermentation is produced by small invisible organisms which could be destroyed by rapid heating. Joseph Lister, a Scottish surgeon, read Pasteur's reports and realised the importance of keeping the hospital environment free of these small organisms today known as bacteria. After experimenting with various chemicals he settled on carbolic acid as an antiseptic; it was 20 years before his antiseptic techniques were widely adopted. The work of Pasteur and a German doctor, Robert Koch, later led to development of vaccines against anthrax, rabies and cholera. These advances laid the foundation for the science of bacteriology.

In 1895 Wilhelm Konrad von Röntgen discovered X-rays while studying the effects of cathode rays. The efficiency of the printing industry had reached a peak. Röntgen published his work on 28 December 1895, and a month later *The Lancet* published an X-ray photograph of a human hand taken in London. Radiography became a discipline, and the value of X-rays in diagnosis was rapidly recognised worldwide.

The 20th century

The end of the 19th century saw dramatic changes in families. Whereas previously a woman could expect to lose over half of her children in their first year of life, by the end of the century she could expect most to survive. Many, supported by the rising feminist movement, began to demand birth-control. For many years only the simplest forms of contraceptives were available, and intra-uterine devices were only available to a very few. Oral contraceptives came on the market in the 1960s and sterilisation became a simple and relatively painless operation.

By the early 20th century professional medical care was much more widely available. Patients could be protected from infections by vaccination, and accidental injuries could be dealt with surgically. Nevertheless, few effective drugs existed. Probably the most important were quinine, morphine, digitalis and aspirin. The first three had been available for several hundred years, and the fourth did not require a prescription.

The pharmacological revolution began in Germany with Paul Ehrlich, a chemist. In 1910 he produced a substance called salvarsan, an effective remedy for syphilis. Alexander Fleming's discovery of penicillin at St Mary's Hospital in London followed in 1928. Antibiotics were the most important drugs to be added to the doctor's armoury in the 20th century. With the advent of penicillin, mortality from pneumonia in the United Sates fell from around 50% to approximately 5%.

There followed the introduction of barbiturates, other sedatives and tranquillisers. The science of endocrinology (study of hormones) began at the start of the 20th century and led to the use of insulin to treat diabetes. Cortisone, isolated just after the Second World War, proved to be vital in treating conditions such as rheumatoid arthritis and asthma. Vaccines were introduced against tetanus, diphtheria, tuberculosis and poliomyelitis. The importance of vitamin deficiencies and their correction were recognised. The World Health Organisation (WHO) was established in 1948 and furthered progress in eradicating infectious diseases worldwide. In 1948, the National Health Service (NHS) was established in Britain. Provision of state support for the sick, elderly and disabled helped lessen poverty and minimise the economic consequences of illness.

In 1962, James Watson and Francis Crick, scientists in Cambridge, shared a Nobel Prize for elucidating the structure of deoxyribonucleic acid (DNA) and the discipline of molecular biology was born. The Human Genome Project is the most ambitious scientific venture since the Apollo project to land men on the moon. The 21st century waits to discover whether it will fulfil its hope of liberation from cancer, heart disease, auto-immune diseases such as rheumatoid arthritis, and some psychiatric illnesses.

Current and future challenges include preventing heart disease, cancer, obesity and industrial hazards in developed countries, managing chronic illnesses, and dealing effectively with threats from global warming. Global pandemics of infectious disease, once thought consigned to history, have re-surfaced. According to

UNAIDS and WHO figures, around 37.2 million adults and 2.3 million children were infected with the human immunodeficiency virus (HIV) by the end of 2006, with sub-Saharan Africa more heavily affected than any other region of the world.[12] Highly contagious diseases such as avian influenza are readily spread by international air travel. Water shortages, air pollution and climate change present further challenges.

Conclusions

From this brief historical outline several principles emerge. The distinction between orthodox medicine and CAM therapies is not always sharply defined. In the accounts of ancient civilisations and their practice of medicine we see the origins of many of the CAM therapies practised today, including Chinese herbal medicine, acupuncture and Ayurvedic medicine. Religion and medicine have always been associated. The church has for a number of reasons allied itself with orthodox medicine in the past, and intellectual and religious debates over the validity of alternative remedies did not originate in the 21st century.

Throughout history the sick have had recourse to practitioners of orthodox medicine as well as to spiritual leaders and 'folk medicine'. We can therefore distinguish between two types of CAM: those which are based on harmless and sometimes useful folklore, and those with a definite spiritual, or religious significance. As we shall see later, some forms of CAM therapies may be regarded as belonging to either one or to both groups, depending on one's viewpoint. While from an economic and scientific perspective it may be important to eliminate ineffective therapies based on folklore alone, it is generally not these that cause most concern to Christians. Rather, those practices with a specific spiritual significance are the most worrying. There are many reasons why, in a supposedly 'scientific' age, such approaches are becoming more widely established, and these will be considered in the next chapter.

It is clear that the health of our society depends also on significant contributions from those outside the medical profession, including social benefactors and governments. The role of the environment and communities in promoting health is a theme we will return to in later chapters. Clearly, the value of scientific research and the importance of interaction between clinicians and non-clinical scientists must never be underestimated. It is also evident that international exchange of ideas has long influenced medical practices in this small island, and the current popularity of CAM therapies with their origins in far flung corners of the world is a contemporary example of this phenomenon.

Finally, it is clear that orthodox medicine does not have a monopoly on the truth, and current assumptions, however firmly based on the best evidence available at the time, may later be shown to be incorrect. Opinions based upon practical knowledge cannot always be lightly dismissed, and Christians must realise that orthodox medicine does not always have all the answers. The medical profession must admit this when appropriate and continue to widen its horizons of knowledge.

References

1. Margotta R. *An Illustrated History of Medicine.* UK: Hamlyn, 1968
2. Lyons A, Petrucelli R. *Medicine: An Illustrated History.* USA: Abradale Press, 1987
3. Wiseman D. *Medicine in the Old Testament World* (see especially select bibliography) in *Medicine and the Bible.* Ed Palmer B. UK: CMF/Paternoster Press, 1986
4. Coleman V. *The Story of Medicine.* UK: Robert Hale, 1985
5. Ed Porter R. *The Cambridge Illustrated History of Medicine.* UK: Cambridge University Press, 1996
6. Emery A, Emery M. *Medicine and Art.* UK: Royal Society of Medicine Press Ltd, 2006
7. Herodotus II.77
8. Leviticus 19:31; 20:6,27
9. John 9:1-7
10. Luke 13:1-5
11. Larner C. *Healing in Pre-Industrial Britain* in *Alternative Medicine in Britain.* Ed Saks, M. UK: Oxford University Press, 1992
12. www.avert.org accessed November 2007

For reflection on your own or for discussion in a small group

1. What can we learn from history about disease?
2. What factors influence a society's views of disease?
3. How are treatments for disease developed?
4. What factors outside the remit of medical practice contribute to a society's health?

3

Why CAM?

Cured yesterday of my disease, I died last night of my physician.
Matthew Prior. *The Remedy Worse than the Disease*

News about him [Jesus] spread… people brought to him all who were ill
with various diseases, those suffering severe pain, the demon-possessed,
those having seizures, and the paralysed, and he healed them.
Matthew 4:24

In this chapter I explore some of the reasons for the recent surge of
interest in CAM in Western nations. To assess what an intelligent
response to CAM should be, it is not enough to note the statistics. We
should also have some idea of what makes it so attractive. Walk down
a typical high street in a prosperous city on a busy working day in
Britain and you are likely to come across at least one if not several
retail outlets offering natural remedies, herbal treatments, dietary
supplements, acupuncture, massage, reflexology, osteopathy and
often more. With the publicity comes the implied promise of better
health, and perhaps more importantly, enhanced well-being. Why are
these approaches generating such interest and financial investment?

Medical progress

Greater expectations
As we saw in the last chapter, modern medicine, including surgery
and anaesthetics, has dramatically altered outcomes for a range of
medical and surgical conditions, resulting in a significantly altered
age distribution for the population. The following figures illustrate
some of the changes.[1-3] Life expectancy at birth in 1840 in England

and Wales was 40 years; by 2005 it had risen to 77 years for men and 81 years for women. Infant deaths (deaths in the first year of life) in the UK in 1870 were 150 per 1,000 live births; by 2005 they had fallen to 5 per 1,000. In 2005 just 36 women died during pregnancy, childbirth and the puerperium in England and Wales. In 1961 only 16 million people in the UK population were aged 50 or over; by 2005 that figure had risen by 27% to 20.3 million.

To imagine the conditions prevalent in Britain in the 19th century we have to turn to famine or war-ravaged countries, where today we see disease claiming many lives on a widespread scale. Alternatively we gain glimpses of life in Europe in the early 20th century by reading contemporary accounts, such as Thomas Mann's description of a tuberculosis sanatorium.[4] Lewis Thomas gives an idea of the revolution in medicine in North America afforded by new technology developed in the 1920s, and the resulting changes which affected patients and doctors alike.[5]

Modern medicine is thus powerful and effective, and seems likely to become more so. The 'miracles' of modern medicine are now largely taken for granted. Patients often assume the availability of 'high-tech' treatments. A patient with newly-diagnosed angina may discuss by-pass surgery or indeed heart transplantation in much the same way as angina medication. A patient with cancer may assume that chemotherapy offers long term, disease-free survival. These patients are understandably anxious, so they naturally search for the most effective treatment, but it is noteworthy that their expectations, quite alien from those of even our grandparents, have been raised very substantially.

So where do these expectations come from? To some extent the medical profession is responsible for creating them. In our enthusiasm over all that modern medicine has to offer, and in our desire to ensure that no-one will miss out, doctors have boldly and confidently publicised their achievements. In the last 20 years, quick to take advantage of a news story, journalists have seized on every new development. The results of successes (and failures) are published in newspapers, television programmes and on the internet. In this country and overseas it is now commonplace for the latest studies reported in the *British Medical Journal*, *The Lancet* and other international medical journals to be discussed on radio and television programmes. The public is better informed than ever before, and expects consistent, measurable results from the medical profession.

Greater disappointment

Our well-informed public, with high expectations of all that modern medicine can offer, is particularly susceptible to disappointment. As outlined below, some of the most pressing problems faced by conventional medicine are the unintended consequences of its success. There are at least three major causes of disenchantment: chronic disease, iatrogenic illnesses and ethical dilemmas.

Chronic disease

Chronic disease presents a significant challenge in Western societies in the 21st century. Despite great achievements in the 20th century, especially in treating infectious diseases and acute surgical problems, conventional medicine still has few effective remedies for long-term illnesses. Indeed, as more of the population survive acute diseases such as pneumonia and appendicitis, more people live to develop chronic conditions, such as heart disease and cancer.

The leading causes of death in Western and Eastern Europe are currently ischaemic heart disease, cerebrovascular disease and lung cancer. However, assuming that research into these conditions will improve survival in the future, a greater proportion of the population will in turn survive to become older, with a consequent rise in the prevalence of dementia. The impact of an illness is thus not only measured by its effect on life expectancy, but also on quality of life. Depression is a scourge of Western societies, causing a greater loss of quality adjusted life years (QALYs) than almost any other illness. Around 15-20% of the population will experience an episode of major depression during their lives; women being more prone to the condition than men. For various reasons the disease is frequently overlooked and inadequately treated.

In most cases doctors are unable to offer cures for common conditions such as asthma, recurrent back pain, epilepsy, diabetes, migraine, dementia and recurrent depression. Where striking advances have been made, such as the use of kidney transplants to treat chronic renal failure, a suitable donor may not be found, or complications such as organ rejection may arise and recovery may be incomplete.

The absence of cures for chronic disease has been compounded in the past by the generally recognised, although often ignored fact, that solving acute health care problems is commonly regarded as being more prestigious. Research into such areas has therefore historically attracted more ambitious physicians and greater government and research council resources (for example research funding) than has the investigation of chronic illness. The British government's recent emphasis on achieving certain health targets (for example better care for patients with asthma or hypertension) could improve this situation. However, long-term significant improvements require increased funding for research, not merely more structured clinical practice aimed at meeting clinical targets. If funding is not available, research into prevention and better treatments will cease and a generation of new doctors will not be attracted into these fields.

Iatrogenic illness
Iatrogenic illnesses are those caused by drugs or procedures used to treat the underlying condition. At the time of writing well-publicised examples include hospital-acquired infections, notably from methicillin-resistant *Staphylococcus aureus* (MRSA), and antibiotic-induced diarrhoea resulting from *Clostridium difficile* infection. In 2004 the UK National Audit Office (NAO) published data showing that the UK had among the highest levels of MRSA bloodstream infections (bacteraemias) in Europe.[6] At any one time the NAO concluded that 9% of hospital patients have an infection caught in hospital and that there are at least 300,000 hospital acquired infections a year. These are estimated to cost the NHS around £1 billion a year and potentially prolong hospital stay by an average of 11 days. No doubt iatrogenic illnesses will continue to present a challenge to overstretched health services even when MRSA and antibiotic-induced diarrhoea have been dealt with.

Some iatrogenic conditions are drug-induced. Medication errors are an increasingly reported phenomenon. It has been estimated that the annual cost of drug-related morbidity and mortality is nearly $177 billion in the United States[7], while the UK National Patient Safety Agency reported in 2006 that over 40,000 medication errors arise per year in the NHS.[8] These figures are inevitably an underestimate since not all errors are reported. Although most caused no harm, 15% caused a low degree of harm and 5% caused moderate or severe harm.

With the widespread use of potent drugs with potentially hazardous side-effects, patients are becoming increasingly aware of their possible risks. CAM therapies may therefore appear attractive because they are promoted as offering 'natural' and supposedly safe remedies. As we shall see later, this is nevertheless sometimes a fallacy, and one which should be exposed to public scrutiny.

Ethical dilemmas

The ingenuity of modern medicine has created a raft of new ethical dilemmas hitherto undreamt of, especially in the field of reproductive medicine. *In vitro* fertilisation (IVF) provides just one example. The vexed question of ownership of eggs fertilised and frozen for storage, the complex issues surrounding surrogate motherhood, and questions around our ability to screen embryos for genetic defects or to perform prenatal sex determination, have all arisen from developments in IVF. Gene therapy, effective life-support systems and transplant surgery engender further questions. A new field, that of bioethics, is expanding rapidly, alongside the establishment of national bioethics commissions in a number of countries.

The issue of rising expenditure on healthcare in developed nations, currently around 15% of gross national product in the US, is another area of controversy. Healthcare rationing, whether explicit or concealed, is of necessity universal, but nevertheless highly contentious.

It is clear that Western populations are not prepared to leave such ethical issues in the hands of politicians, scientists or physicians alone; public debate is called for. Inevitably some have consequently become disillusioned with the benefits of modern medicine.

'My doctor seems remote'

When infections such as bubonic plague, typhus, tuberculosis and syphilis were usually lethal despite all the doctor's efforts, the doctor often had nothing to offer the patient for palliation, let alone cure. Consequently physicians learnt to give a sympathetic word and a handshake to victims sometimes shunned by friends or relatives. Physical contact imparted confidence to patients, and was developed to a fine art in the techniques of organ palpation and use of the stethoscope. Very often the doctor was present at the patient's death, providing some comfort to both the patient and the family. The physician thus performed a role as a trusted friend, usually alongside the local religious leader, or priest in Christian countries.

Today's modern technology renders such a role difficult to fulfil. Contemporary medicine offers a machine model of the human body, and healthcare professionals in many fields have become expert technicians rather than friends or healers. Sophisticated equipment such as computers, scanners, endoscopes and lasers are altering clinical practice beyond recognition and absorb much of doctors' attention. Patients are often treated in hospital, in unfamiliar and clinical surroundings. Those in coronary care or high dependency units have their rest disrupted by noisy monitors. Those with terminal cancer receiving palliative care on general wards are at risk of being overlooked by busy junior doctors, for whom such contact may be both uncomfortable and time-consuming. Elderly patients do not always receive the help they need at mealtimes and their dignity is not always preserved. If patients, friends and families do not feel understood, respected and cared for, it should come as no surprise if they seek different sources of support.

In the UK, the structure and organisation of the UK National Health Service (NHS) itself may also be partly to blame. The proportion of hospital employees directly involved in patient care has fallen since its inception, while the percentage of administrative staff has risen dramatically. Twentieth century hospitals were often built as impersonal multi-storey blocks without regard to aesthetics. In a 19th century hospital the patients' ward was the most important part of the building, whereas in a modern centre of excellence, for whatever good reasons, wards occupy only about 20% of the space. Florence Nightingale was an early proponent of the view that the physical environment afforded by a hospital could itself be therapeutic or otherwise. She wrote: 'I have seen the most acute suffering produced from a patient not being able to see out of a window. I shall never forget the rapture of fever patients over a bunch of brightly coloured flowers. People say the effect is only the mind. It is no such thing. The effect is on the body too.'[9]

'My doctor is too busy'

Increasing day case care means that many patients spend under 24 hours in hospital. Junior doctors and consultants alike have limited opportunity to listen to patients' concerns. Hospital consultants are busier in other areas, with increased roles in administration and hospital audit. They may be required to comply with goals set by hospital managers, for example to reduce outpatient waiting times. Such goals are often very desirable, as anyone who has waited in an outpatients department knows well, but they put pressure on time available for consultations. It can therefore be a challenge even for the most caring and conscientious doctor working in such situations to devote adequate time to a patient's worries. An anxious and frightened patient may understandably feel let down.

Social change

Single households
Since the 1960s there has been a significant increase in the proportion of households containing people living alone and single parents with dependant children.[10] There are several reasons for this. Increased life-expectancy, itself the product of modern medicine, means that a greater proportion of households contain only one elderly person. Increased mobility has caused more people to leave their home town or village to live and work among strangers. Finally, changes in society's values have resulted in a rise in the number of households containing singles and divorcees. This often means reduced contact with family or friends, and those living alone may not find support in times of illness quite so readily. Some may turn instead to their general practitioner for support. If a sympathetic ear and time for listening are not forthcoming, they may more readily turn to a CAM therapist.

Rejection of religion
Between 1980 and 2000 the Church of England saw a drop of 27% in church membership.[11] It is estimated that only around 7.5% of the British population attend church regularly today. Non-churchgoers are extremely unlikely to know their local vicar or lay members of the church, who might previously have provided comfort in times of illness.

In a society where belief in medicine has largely replaced a belief in God, many doctors are failing to fulfil the role previously played by church ministers. People no longer trust a God they do not believe in with the outcome of their illness, and many are desperate. Those whom modern medicine can neither cure nor comfort will turn just about anywhere else in their quest for help and encouragement.

A multicultural society
Immigration is not a new phenomenon in Britain. It has been estimated that even in the 18th century there were 20,000 black people living in this country, and in the 19th century large numbers of Irish immigrants entered England, particularly during the potato famines in the 1840s.

In the 1950s, immigration from the Commonwealth, particularly from the Caribbean, was actively encouraged in order to meet labour shortages. Over 80% of teenagers of West Indian origin were born in Britain, showing that these immigrants have settled in this country and had families. Asians, Indians and Pakistani nationals have for the last 200 years or so comprised the majority of other ethnic minorities, but a wave of immigration from Eastern Europe following EU expansion in the 21st century is changing the composition of the British population once again. No-one can doubt that we live in a multi-racial society.

This can contribute to the increasing demand for CAM therapies in several ways. Immigrants recently arrived from overseas may have different expectations of doctors and medicine. They may expect time and contact with the physician and may be less familiar with modern technology. They may collectively bring CAM remedies with them. A particularly striking example of this is seen in the widespread market for Chinese remedies, particularly for eczema. Finally, the first generation of settlers at least is more likely to belong to less affluent sections of the community. This group will thereby be subject to the inequalities in health outlined below.

The gap between rich and poor
In many societies, the lower down the social scale individuals find themselves, the less healthy they are and the shorter their life expectancy. The reasons will differ between countries but the following examples illustrate some of them.

Where medical care has to be paid for directly by the patient to the doctor or hospital, those who are poorer will tend to avoid seeking medical help if at all possible. This will often mean that problems thought by the patient and his or her family to be less serious will be neglected. In addition, where receiving medical care involves travelling some distance, for instance to a specialised hospital, those on lower incomes may not feel able to continue receiving such treatment because of the prohibitive cost of public transport.

Certain occupations have health risks associated with them. An obvious example is coal mining. Traditionally such occupations are taken up by less affluent members of society, who then become more likely to develop lung disease.

Families on poorer incomes in any country tend to have restricted access to the best education provided by that country. The cumulative result of generations of poor education is a diminished understanding of the causes of disease and measures for prevention.

In communities without prospect of employment or improved living standards, even simple health messages promoted by the government may fall on deaf ears because of understandable apathy and cynicism.

Finally, low income has a direct adverse effect on diet and therefore nutrition. A lowered consumption of fresh meat, fish, vegetables and fruit, which in Western countries tend to be more expensive than so-called 'junk foods' high in fat and sugar, has well-documented adverse consequences on health.

When the NHS was founded in 1948, it was based on the principles that medical care in Britain should be paid for by indirect taxation, and that all should have access to medical care regardless of income. Nevertheless, there remains a significant gap between the health of the poor and the rich in Britain today. It was highlighted by the Report of the Working Group on Inequalities in Health (known as the Black Report) in 1980 and has been confirmed by independent reports since. Notable exemptions from the principle of free medical care are prescription charges and the fees charged by dentists and opticians.

Of greater concern, however, is that differences in mortality (death rates) and morbidity (sickness rates) between the rich and the poor have continued to increase since 1980. As chronic diseases now constitute a greater proportion of all conditions in the UK, the relationship between mortality and morbidity is weaker than previously. Therefore studying death rates alone may not yield a true reflection of health in this country today. The NHS is thus failing to ensure equality of medical care throughout society and many are consequently disillusioned with conventional medicine.

A further inequality in society is the use of the health service by men and women. Women are the biggest users of healthcare facilities, reflecting their responsibilities in child-bearing and child-rearing. Many have taken up this issue and 'well-women clinics' attempt to address it. However, women remain at present poorly represented among the higher ranks of the medical profession. Some women may therefore seek to control their own medical care by turning to CAM practitioners who may not carry such a patriarchal or paternalistic image.

What does CAM offer?

Time
Mostly working in private practice, CAM practitioners take more time. They offer time to listen to patients and explain their problem

to them. An average first session with a CAM practitioner lasts for one hour, at least twice the time generally afforded for a first consultation with a hospital consultant. Time invested by a practitioner communicates care and compassion to the patient, and may also provide the patient with a sense of greater control over his or her future.

Touch

The traditional handshake and an arm around the shoulder are for various reasons less common in modern consultations. In contrast, CAM practitioners offer an increased amount of touch in a 'low-tech' environment.

Without exerting any specific effect on the disease, touch expresses involvement and can make people feel better, which is what most patients want. Many CAM therapies provide a degree of physical contact and thereby reassurance not afforded by conventional medications. Various forms of massage, and aromatherapy, are examples of CAM therapies which provide substantial physical contact with the patient.

Trust

CAM practitioners tend to have very good communications skills which put patients at ease.[12] CAM consultations not only take more time, they are often more thorough and detailed than conventional medical consultations. CAM practitioners tend to include active listening techniques and show interest in the whole patient's life, not just in their physical health. Such factors are likely to contribute to higher levels of patient satisfaction with their treatment, particularly when conventional medicine offers busy practitioners in an understaffed NHS.

Zollmann and Vickers[13] have suggested that CAM consultations add value in terms of attention to personality and experience, greater patient involvement and choice, more hope resulting from a holistic approach, and a more human experience of healthcare. In addition they point out that CAM often specialises in dealing with ill-defined symptoms that conventional medicine may be unable or unwilling to tackle.

It is well known that the 'gut feeling' of either the doctor or the patient about a particular treatment is not always a good guide to how effective that treatment really is. This is partly because both doctors and patients tend to be biased in favour of treatment, and partly because of the placebo phenomenon.

'Placebo' literally means 'I shall please'. Originally a placebo was a pharmacologically inert compound prepared to satisfy the patient's desire for treatment rather than specifically to treat his or her disease. Some placebos might have pharmacological activity not specifically effective for the illness, an example being a vitamin preparation given as a 'tonic' to a patient who is not vitamin-deficient.

One third of all people given an inert compound to relieve a particular symptom will report relief of that symptom.[14] This phenomenon is known as the 'placebo effect', and it depends on various factors. An early study showed that red placebo tablets were more effective in relieving pain than blue ones, and these in turn were more effective than green tablets.[15] A more recent study has shown that the placebo response can be modified by the attitude of the healthcare staff, the size and shape as well as the colour of the medication, and whether it is given by mouth or by injection.[16] Authoritative, kind healthcare staff augment the placebo response, and injections are more effective than tablets. The importance of the placebo effect is emphasised by studies showing that placebos can be as effective as active treatments, and that for psychological disorders, particularly depression, pill placebos are nearly as effective as active medications. Furthermore, psychological placebos, if well-designed, can be as effective as accepted psychotherapeutic approaches in treating depression.[17]

The confidence of both the doctor and the patient in a particular drug or treatment, as well as the patient's trust in the practitioner, can thus profoundly affect the patient's response to treatment. This should not surprise us; much early medicine consisted of rituals which were effective to some extent if the patient believed in them.

Current technology in medicine is removing the placebo effect. Computers, scanners and biochemical analysers can provide diagnostic tests and be used to deliver and control therapy. If doctors, nurses and other healthcare professionals have insufficient time to impart confidence, the only area where the placebo effect will still play a role is in the colour, shape and size of tablets and the route of administration.

CAM practitioners restore some of the art and indeed mystery of medicine, and this may reinforce belief in the practitioner's skills. Where conventional medicine has failed, a CAM practitioner's confident arguments for the cause and remedy of the disease may sound very convincing.

Sometimes it really works

In some cases, CAM offers effective treatment, as the following two examples illustrate. Osteopathy was until recently regarded by much of the medical profession as potentially hazardous and probably ineffective. Now it is increasingly offered by general practitioners alongside conventional medicine. Some studies have shown that patients derive greater benefit from osteopathy than from other forms of treatment, particularly for chronic low back pain, and the Osteopaths Act passed in 1993 provided for regulation of all osteopathic practitioners. Osteopathy is set to become part of future mainstream medicine. There is now some evidence that St John's Wort (*hypericum*) contains an active drug which is effective in the treatment of mild to moderate depression, and that it may exert its therapeutic effect in the same way as one group of conventional antidepressants, the selective serotonin re-uptake inhibitors.

Michael Hyland, Professor of Health Psychology at the University of Plymouth, believes that CAM can sometimes be effective in chronic illness. He points out that modern Western medicine assumes the body to function like a mechanical system, such as a clock, computer or jumbo jet.[18] This model presupposes that disease results from a specific error in the system due to a precise cause. Treatment is thus given to correct that particular fault. In situations where there is such a precise cause, an example being invasion of the bloodstream by an infectious organism, Western medicine has in general been very successful.

In contrast, many CAM therapists regard the body as an ecological system, analogous to the environmental ecological systems we increasingly recognise. Illness is thought to result from an imbalance in the system, an example being an imbalance between yin and yang. Since the cause may be considered to be multi-factorial, treatment is directed at the whole person, may not be disease-specific, and often comprises several treatments given simultaneously.

Professor Hyland argues that orthodox medical practitioners may need to revisit the somewhat narrow modern Western models of disease and entertain the possibility that the body in many cases functions as a series of networks. He defines networks as systems which can do lots of things simultaneously. Examples of networks are the brain, our hormonal system, and the immune system. He then defines network pathologies as those which arise from errors in the relationship between parts throughout the system, and which lead to failure of normal self-regulation. From this he draws the conclusion that some effective CAM treatments work at the network level, and involve lifestyle factors, psychosocial and nutritional influences which are often neglected by orthodox practitioners.

A spiritual dimension

The decline in interest in mainstream religion and Christianity in this country does not necessarily mean that people don't want spiritual support in times of illness. It merely means that many have turned to other sources. We have already noted the link between disease and spiritual beliefs. Now that modern Western medicine no longer offers answers as to the significance of the illness or the threat of death, some CAM therapies may offer a spiritual dimension not found in the NHS. Professor Hyland suggests it is no coincidence that it is individuals with a high level of spirituality who turn to CAM and find benefit in CAM approaches.

It is precisely because some CAM therapies *do* work that so many of them can be attractive to the desperate patient. They are also relatively difficult to evaluate scientifically, making it difficult to distinguish fact from fiction. How we might begin to do this is the subject of the next chapter.

Controversy is not new

Before proceeding to the next chapter, it is important to recall that dissatisfaction with the medical profession is not new. Doctors have always had to contend with criticism and complaints. Given the factors outlined above it is therefore not surprising that doctors today are increasingly unable to meet their patients' expectations, despite the dramatic therapeutic progress made in some fields.

References

1. Office of Health Economics. *Compendium of Health Statistics*. London UK: 8th Edition, 1992
2. *Mortality Statistics. Series DH2 no 32 and DH3 no 38*. www.statistics.gov.uk accessed June 2007
3. Economic & Social Research Council. www.esrcsocietytoday.co.uk accessed June 2007
4. Mann T. *The Magic Mountain*. UK: Penguin Books, 1924
5. Thomas L. *The Youngest Science*. UK: Oxford University Press, 1985
6. *Improving patient care by reducing the risk of hospital acquired infection: a progress report*. National Audit Office HC 876 Session 2003-4: 14 July 2004
7. Riedl M, Casillas A. Adverse drug reactions: types and treatment options. *American Family Physician* 2003; 68:1781-1789
8. Bosely S. *The Guardian* 11 August 2006
9. Nightingale F. *Notes on nursing: what it is and what it is not*. New York: Dover publications, 1969
10. Abercrombie N, Warde A. *Families and Households* in *Contemporary British Society*. UK: Polity Press, 1988
11. Furlong M. *The Church of England: the state it's in*. UK: Stoughton, 2000
12. The House of Lords Select Committee on Science & Technology Sixth Report. London UK: 21 November 2000
13. Zollman C, Vickers A. ABC of Complementary Medicine: Complementary Medicine & the Patient. *BMJ* 1999; 319: 1486-89
14. Graham-Smith D, Aronson J. *Oxford Textbook of Clinical Pharmacology and Drug Therapy*. UK: Oxford University Press, 1984
15. Huskisson E. Simple analgesics for arthritis. *BMJ* 1974; iv: 196-200
16. Miller F, Rosenstein D. The nature and power of the placebo effect. *J Clinical Epidemiology* 2006; 59:331-335
17. Wampold B *et al*. The story of placebo effects in medicine: evidence in context. *J Clin Psychol* 2007; 63:379-390
18. Hyland M. The intelligent body. *New Scientist* 2001; 170: 32-33

For reflection on your own or for discussion in a small group

1. Have you ever attended a busy NHS clinic as a patient at a hospital where no-one knows you?
2. Have you ever consulted a CAM practitioner?
3. Compare your experiences in each case:
   a) how long did you wait to be seen?
   b) what did each cost (fees, time, travel, etc)
   c) how were you greeted by the receptionist and/or nurse?
   d) how long did each consultation last?
   e) how did you feel as you left?
4. How can healthcare practitioners help to make patients more comfortable with the NHS care they receive? Would you consider getting personally involved to make your local hospital a more welcoming environment?
5. Should the church and/or Christian communities support those outside the church who are ill? If so, how can they approach this challenge?

4

CAM: some challenges

The wisdom of the prudent is to give thought to their ways. Proverbs 14:8

There are two equal and opposite errors into which our race can fall about the devils. One is to disbelieve in their existence. The other is to believe, and to feel an excessive and unhealthy interest in them. They themselves are equally pleased by both errors.   CS Lewis. *The Screwtape Letters*

In this chapter we will look at some of the evidence for genuine risks associated with the various therapeutic practices included under the CAM umbrella. This is necessary before deciding how best to approach them.

At this point it is helpful to classify the main types of CAM currently practised. We have already seen that there is no unifying concept underlying these therapies; they are merely grouped together because they lie outside the scope of conventional medicine. Their diversity of approach is a challenge to classification, as is evident by the fact that they are so often merely listed alphabetically. Nevertheless, even a simple classification helps us to understand both the rationale and potential hazards associated with each one. More information on individual therapies is given in chapter seven.

Since the CMF published *Alternative Medicine: Helpful or Harmful?*, several classifications of CAM therapies have been proposed. The US-based National Center for Complementary and Alternative Medicine groups CAM therapies into five domains. The first comprises alternative medical systems, which transcend all the other four domains and may have developed in Western or non-Western cultures. Examples are homoeopathic and naturopathic medicine, which developed in the West, and traditional Chinese medicine and Ayuverdic medicine which developed outside Western culture. The second domain is that of mind-body medicine, which includes meditation and therapies involving dance, art and music. The third domain consists of biologically based therapies, such as herbs, foods and vitamins. The fourth domain comprises manipulative therapies such as osteopathy and chiropractic, and the fifth comprises energy therapies. These can be of two types; for example Reiki, which aims to influence unproven energy fields surrounding a particular subject, and unconventional use of electromagnetic fields. This classification has the advantage of providing a clear overall introduction to each approach, but does not highlight particular aspects of alternative medical systems.

A classification of CAM has also been proposed by the House of Lords Select Committee on Science & Technology, which describes three groups.[1] The first group comprises the five most commonly practised disciplines, namely osteopathy and chiropractic, both regulated by Acts of Parliament, acupuncture, herbal medicine and homoeopathy. The House of Lords concluded that therapies in this group claim to have an individual diagnostic approach, and are regarded as the five most significant therapies by CAM advocates. The second group comprises CAM therapies which are often used to complement orthodox medicine but do not profess to offer a diagnosis. They include aromatherapy, the Alexander Technique, massage, counselling, hypnotherapy, reflexology, shiatsu, and meditation. The third group comprises CAM therapies which claim to offer diagnostic information and often embrace philosophies independent of scientific principles. Two sub-groups are distinguished. The first includes long-established and traditional systems of healthcare such as Ayurvedic medicine and traditional Chinese medicine, while the second includes other CAM therapies with no evidence base, such as crystal therapy, iridology, radionics and kinesiology. The clear advantages of this classification are that it highlights issues of popularity, professional regulation, evidence base and underlying philosophy, and it is thus eminently practical and a useful aide-mémoire. A possible downside is that it might lead to unjustified assumptions. As an example, the inclusion of certain CAM therapies in the first group might give them an apparent credibility not warranted by current evidence, while wisdom from traditional systems of healthcare might be dismissed.

In *Alternative Medicine: Helpful or Harmful?*, I also grouped CAM therapies into three groups. However, this was based on their method of delivery, whether external (physical), internal or psychic. Using this classification, external or physical treatments involve massage or manipulation. Examples include acupuncture, the Alexander Technique, aromatherapy, chiropractic, osteopathy, kinesiology, reflexology and shiatsu. Internal treatments involve taking medicines (sometimes rather attractively called elixirs, oils or infusions) internally, usually by mouth, but sometimes as enemas. Examples include Bach flower remedies, herbalism and homoeopathy. Psychic treatments include CAM therapies which are psychological, paranormal or spiritual in origin, the paranormal making use of forces not recognised by natural laws. Examples include crystal therapy, hypnotherapy, radionics and transcendental meditation. Some treatments encompass more than one of these concepts.

It is clear from the above that there is no single perfect classification for what is a very diverse group of therapeutic approaches. Nevertheless my original grouping may still serve the purposes of this book, aimed at a general Christian readership likely to be particularly interested in safety and in the philosophies underlying CAM. All three classifications have their merits and readers should adopt whichever they find most helpful. A noticeable feature of many CAM therapies is that as a group they make considerable use of physical and 'spiritual' treatments. In contrast, orthodox medicine generally relies on taking medicine or performing surgical procedures. This has implications for the types of hazards which can result from CAM.

The risks of CAM

According to the main emphasis of any particular remedy, potential hazards can also be classified as being physical, directly affecting physical functioning of one or more organs in the body, or psychic, when the effects may involve more subtle effects on people's mental state, beliefs or psychological experiences.

Physical hazards

One of the most misleading statements often made about herbal remedies is that because they are 'natural' they cannot cause harm. The following examples frankly contradict this claim.

Already in 1994 there were reported to be over 600 clinics offering traditional Chinese medicine in the United Kingdom.[2] Current figures are likely to be higher; furthermore Chinese remedies are now readily available over the internet. Chinese herbal remedies are often recommended for eczema, a distressing skin condition frequently affecting children. It can cause misery through constant itching, sleepless nights and skin disfigurement resulting in social isolation. Chinese herbal remedies have produced dramatic improvement in some patients in whom the condition was previously resistant to orthodox treatment. Parents are therefore understandably under considerable pressure to try such treatments when mainstream medicine has failed to bring relief. However, there has long been concern about the safety of these remedies. There is considerable evidence that they may contain both uncharacterised compounds with serious and poorly documented side-effects, such as heavy metals, and potent conventional pharmacological agents with well-known hazards.

The Medicines and Healthcare Products Regulatory Agency (MHRA) is the UK government agency responsible for ensuring that medicines are effective and acceptably safe. It notes that adulteration of both traditional Chinese medicines and unlicensed Ayurvedic medicines with mercury, lead and arsenic is a significant international problem.[3] These metals and their salts pose a serious public health risk. In addition to nausea, vomiting and abdominal pain, convulsions, paralysis and even coma can result from their ingestion. US surveys in 2004 showed that 20% of all Ayurvedic medicines in the Boston area contained potentially harmful levels of lead, mercury and arsenic. In December that year the MHRA was alerted to reports from Hong Kong that a product called Tik Dak Win, from the Ng Chung brand, had been found to contain high levels of lead. Some agents, particularly Chinese herbal creams, have been shown repeatedly to contain corticosteroids[4], the potent agents used in mainstream medicine for treating eczema. This is ironic when the public are increasingly questioning the safety of steroids prescribed by mainstream physicians for a variety of conditions, and considering 'natural' herbal treatments as a safer alternative. It is also worrying since application of potent steroids to some sensitive areas, such as the face, can result in thinning of the skin, permanent scarring and severe dermatitis.

In 1999 *The Lancet* reported two UK cases of end-stage renal failure in patients using Chinese herbal remedies containing a plant species, *Aristolochia*, for the treatment of eczema.[5] Aristocholic acids can cause cancer and are associated with a severe form of kidney disease called interstitial nephropathy. In 1993 in Belgium, over 70 cases of renal failure were reported associated with substitution of *Aristolochia* for *Stephania* in a herbal slimming preparation.[6]

Toxicity is not confined to Chinese herbal remedies. Kava-kava, a herbal sedative alleged to have anti-anxiety or calming effects, can cause severe skin rashes, liver toxicity, exacerbation of Parkinson's disease and abnormal movements (including torticollis and painful twisting movements of the trunk).[7-9] Ginkgo biloba, promoted to improve cognitive function and blood flow, inhibits blood clotting and can therefore cause spontaneous bleeding. Several reports have been published of patients who suffered brain haemorrhage while taking this agent[10-12], and ginkgo appears to increase the risk of bleeding when taken with other drugs affecting blood clotting including aspirin, warfarin, clopidogrel (Plavix) and dipyridamole (Persantin).

St John's Wort (*Hypericum perforatum*) is a herb widely promoted as a 'natural' antidepressant, and is commonly prescribed in Germany for anxiety and depression. There are however several case reports of adverse effects in patients taking St John's Wort, including dry mouth, dizziness, confusion, gastrointestinal symptoms, fatigue, increased sensitivity to sunlight manifested by skin rashes and neuropathy (damage to peripheral nerves).[13-16] Furthermore, St John's Wort interacts with a wide variety of conventional therapeutic agents, including cyclosporin, digoxin, theophylline, warfarin, oral contraceptives and orthodox antidepressants. The *British National Formulary*, a leading source of prescribing information for UK doctors, now lists 19 drugs or categories of agents whose actions can be affected by interaction with St John's Wort.[17] In some cases such interactions can be life-threatening.

These examples illustrate at least four problems associated with such remedies.

1. *The ingredients are unknown.* Most herbal products are currently unlicensed, meaning that the ingredients do not have to be declared, and both patients and doctors may be unaware of their contents.
2. *The ingredients may be toxic.* Such treatments may contain drugs used in conventional medicine which are known to have potentially dangerous side-effects. The doses may exceed those usually prescribed by orthodox practitioners.
3. *Contamination may exist.* Since legal requirements for tests of purity and content vary, there may be unrecognised contamination with undesirable substances. These may include other herbs, drugs and various chemicals (for example heavy metals).

4. *The ingredients may interact.* Finally, the active ingredients present in these formulations may interact with orthodox medicines already prescribed for the patient by a medical doctor. Such interactions may have grave consequences.

In response to such concerns, the Medical Toxicology Unit at Guy's & St Thomas' NHS Trust has established a Chinese Medicine Advisory Service providing information to doctors treating patients who have taken these remedies, other herbal remedies or Ayurvedic treatments. An online reporting form is available to document side-effects from herbal remedies; the information is then forwarded to the Committee on Safety of Medicines. The Medical Toxicology Unit website also provides information for patients on herbal remedies, Chinese and Ayurvedic medicine.[18]

Are the risks greater than for orthodox medicine?

It may be argued that many CAM therapies have been used for centuries with few ill effects. The cases given above may represent only exceptional incidents used to increase prejudice within the medical profession against such remedies. Since orthodox medicines can be toxic, why are doctors so concerned about occasional side-effects resulting from the use of herbal remedies?

There are several reasons for serious concern. Side-effects resulting from these remedies may be unpredictable because ingredients are not listed on the packaging. Even if they are listed there may be little medical experience of such agents or of their interaction with orthodox remedies. Furthermore, there may be unintentional contamination with other harmful substances. Since side-effects are unpredictable, patients cannot be forewarned about them. It again seems ironic that, in the search for greater patient freedom, patients have in fact sometimes taken giant leaps backwards, not forwards. While insisting that they should be better informed with regard to the hazards of modern drugs and surgery, they are risking serious poisoning from substances about which they have either little or no information whatsoever. As discussed in the next chapter, much of the information provided with CAM remedies can be misleading and some of it may be frankly untrue.

Natural does not mean harmless

I am particularly concerned that the public often believes the claim that these remedies are 'natural' and therefore harmless, even if they prove to be ineffective. In the face of inadequate or unpleasant orthodox therapy, the temptation to try them then becomes almost irresistible. The above examples show that 'natural' or herbal remedies can be extremely toxic. Conversely, a significant number of powerful modern drugs have been developed from herbal sources. However, this in no way means that they are harmless, as the following examples illustrate.

Curare is a resin obtained from certain tropical trees. Owing to its ability to cause muscular paralysis and death in high doses it was used by the South American Indians as an arrow poison. Nevertheless, curare derivatives, such as tubocurarine and pancuronium, are now routinely administered during surgical anaesthesia to induce muscle relaxation.

Digitalis was originally isolated from the pretty foxglove of rural England. In 1776 William Withering, a Birmingham physician, described its effectiveness in the treatment of dropsy or ankle swelling, now known to be a feature of some forms of heart disease. He himself had learnt about the usefulness of foxglove leaves from an elderly lady he met while travelling to Shropshire. Today, digitalis remains an important weapon in the treatment of heart disease. It is given to treat irregularities of heart rhythm and to improve the pumping efficiency of the heart. Despite its natural origin, digitalis can be hazardous and its use requires careful monitoring. It can cause fatal irregularities of the heartbeat rhythm at relatively low circulating concentrations. Less severe side-effects include loss of appetite, nausea, vomiting, diarrhoea, confusion, aversion to bright light (photophobia), blurring of vision and disordered perception of colour.

Aspirin is derived from a compound isolated from the graceful willow tree. Its value was highlighted in 1763 by a paper to the Royal Society of Medicine entitled 'An account of the success of the bark of the willow in the cure of the agues'. Its scientific name, salicylate, comes from the Latin name for willow (*salix*). Aspirin has pain-relieving and anti-inflammatory properties and effectively reduces fever. Even in normal doses it causes a small degree of gastro-intestinal bleeding. In prolonged treatment, or in patients with a predisposition to gastro-intestinal bleeding, it may cause life-threatening blood loss. In cases of self-poisoning with aspirin, the subject may develop tinnitus (ringing in the ears), deafness, a high fever with sweating and dehydration, stomach pains, vomiting, gastro-intestinal haemorrhage, reduced blood sugar levels, respiratory disturbances and impaired consciousness.

Morphine, a powerful painkiller, was isolated from the South West Asian poppy (*Papaver somniferum*), an attractive plant with greyish-green leaves and white or red flowers. Morphine relieves severe pain and is widely used in pre-operative medication. It may be used in heart disease and helps suppress coughing. However, the sedative and euphoric effects of morphine and related compounds have led to long-standing worldwide abuse, exemplified in England by opium dens in the 19th century and intravenous heroin addiction in the 21st century. Less alluring side effects include respiratory depression, nausea, vomiting and constipation.

Atropine is a modern drug derived from the deadly nightshade (*Atropa belladonna*). It has a variety of uses which include reduction of secretions prior to surgery, treatment of the very slow pulse which can follow a heart attack, dilating pupils prior to eye examination, relief of airway narrowing in asthma, treatment of Parkinson's disease and prevention of travel sickness. Side-effects include drying of the mouth, blurred vision, constipation, the eye disease glaucoma in susceptible individuals, confusion, restlessness and hallucinations.

I hope I have now convinced the reader that 'natural' remedies are not harmless just because they are isolated from natural sources such as plants. There is no such thing as a 'good' drug or a 'bad' drug. All the drugs discussed above are extremely valuable therapeutic tools and yet may be fatal in overdose. Indeed, if an agent has no side-effects at all it is probably ineffective. The fallacy that 'natural means harmless' is one which all professionals involved in patient education should firmly destroy once and for all.

Spiritual risks

It is obviously difficult to define such risks. However, it does appear that there are effects associated with certain types of CAM therapies, often those where a spiritual element is involved. It is even more difficult to be precise about the extent and nature of such effects. Given that many medical practitioners and some of the public question the existence of the paranormal realm altogether, this is not surprising. Much evidence is anecdotal and is inevitably influenced by personal beliefs.

In his book, *Hard Questions about Health and Healing*, Dr Andrew Fergusson vividly recounts how one of his patients developed worsening and severe headaches necessitating a night time emergency home visit by a GP, a few hours after consulting a spiritual healer.[19] Although not a Christian believer herself, her symptoms resolved instantly with simple prayer.

The late Dr George Smith, general practitioner and dermatologist, reported that some Christians have suffered what one might label spiritual side-effects from involvement in yoga and transcendental meditation. He listed anxiety, depression, fear, lack of Christian assurance, interference with prayer life and Bible reading, and demonic oppression amongst possible hazards, but did not cite specific examples.[20]

Kurt Koch, a Christian theologian, recounts the story of a young man who received treatment from an iridologist and soon afterwards recovered completely from his illness.[21] However, he subsequently noticed that every time he tried to enter a church, sing a hymn or read the Bible, he experienced intense physical pain. As a result he quickly became severely depressed, started abusing drugs and eventually had a complete emotional breakdown. Kurt Koch discerned the effect of the occult in this particular instance, although clearly not all iridologists have an association with the occult.

In the light of such cautionary tales, it is evidently important to examine those CAM therapies which have their origins in the psychic realm.

Some obvious problems

A popular concept in many branches of CAM is that of a 'life force' or 'vital energy' within the body. Christians should be aware that the theme of 'energy' is also the unifying thread running through the diverse dogmas of the New Age movement. Following directly from ancient Chinese beliefs, good health is sometimes said to depend upon a balance between its two components, referred to as 'yin' and 'yang'. Other terms for these 'energies' include naturopathy's 'vital force', 'Mesmer's magnetism', 'cosmic energy', 'universal energy', 'chi life force' and 'biomagnetic'. Many practitioners believe that healing energy can be transmitted directly from one person to another.

Two CAM therapies developed from such beliefs include yoga and transcendental meditation (TM). They are based on Hindu religious philosophy. The purpose of yoga, as taught by Hindu teachers, is to unite the human spirit with Hindu gods by means of various physical postures. Hindu teachers of yoga believe that all yoga is a religious exercise, that each position represents an act of worship to a Hindu god, and that the physical exercises cannot be divorced from spiritual involvement.

For Christians, therefore, it seems clear that practising yoga or TM is not a valid option, since we are to worship the one and only living God. For non-Christians there is a choice, but it would be reasonable for all doctors and patients to be made aware that these are not strictly medical, but religious practices.

The not so obvious problems

It is not always clear when CAM therapies involve spiritual or religious practices. Terms for healing are often used which may sound quite rational, or at least harmless and acceptable to Christians. These include 'massage', 'laying on of hands', 'holistic' and 'wellness'.

In the late 1980s, Jane Gumprecht[22] emphasised an association between healing promoted by the New Age movement and many CAM therapies practised in the USA. A Christian doctor whose parents were enticed into New Age philosophies, she was well qualified to examine the subject. Some of her conclusions are discussed below.

Dr Gumprecht attributed the overwhelming North American emphasis on strenuous exercise to New Age influence. She pointed out that extreme exercise can be hazardous, resulting in sudden death, musculoskeletal injuries and infertility in young women. It is also well known that strenuous exercise leads to euphoria or a 'natural high'. Jane Gumprecht believed that the New Age goal is to promote heightened awareness. One does not necessarily have to accept this view of New Age involvement in order to perceive the nature of the attraction. What makes people devote excessive time and money to strenuous exercise? Is it a morbid fear of illness, a desire to be fashionable, or both?

The Bible certainly emphasises the need to take care of our physical bodies.[23] When considering our priorities it is appropriate to examine our lifestyle to see if anything should be altered. We are well advised to seek medical advice when concerned. Regular exercise, a balanced diet, moderation in alcohol intake and smoking cessation are all wise precautions. For some, depending on their lifestyle, regular gym sessions and taking advice from a personal trainer may be vital in maintaining physical health and a sensible weight, as well as in relieving stress. However, part of the Bible's teaching is that mankind tends to worship what is created (for example, animals or birds, the sun and the stars, money or material possessions) rather than the one God who created these things.[24] Such created things, when they become more important to us than God, are described as idols. If as Christians we pursue the fitness goal obsessively, we may make an idol out of it. This should be apparent to Christians whether or not they regard the promotion of excessive exercise as arising from the New Age movement.

Vegetarianism is considered by some Christians to be an area of concern. Vegetarianism is a major component of Hinduism and the Hare Krishna cult, to name just two movements. The Hindu faith forbids Hindus in India to eat cows because they are sacred. It has been estimated that, were the cows eaten rather than fed, India's food supply problems could be obliterated. Various recently established animal rights groups have embraced the vegetarian theme and some of their literature is steeped in New Age influence, with liberal use of such terms as 'Mother Earth'.

Some Christians point to the Garden of Eden account as supporting a vegetarian lifestyle. A frequently quoted verse is Genesis 1:29, which is used to support the claim. The rationale is that since plant food was given to Adam and Eve, God still intends his people to eat only plant-based food. In the opening chapter of Daniel, Daniel and his companions are apparently commended for consuming only vegetables and water. However, much evidence from the Bible apparently conflicts with the view that vegetarianism is central to the Judeo-Christian tradition. In Genesis 4 Abel pleased God with his livestock offering. In Genesis 9, after the flood, God gave meat to Noah and his family as food. In Genesis 18 Abraham served angelic visitors butter, milk and meat, which they received and ate. In Exodus 16 God sent quail as food for the Israelites. In Leviticus God listed clean and unclean animals, with clean animals designated as appropriate for food. Jesus himself is repeatedly recorded in the Gospels as eating fish, and a later apostolic council commanded Gentile believers to abstain only from meat killed in a certain way. Fortunately for contemporary Christians, in his letter to the Romans Paul stated that dietary teaching is one of those matters on which Christians may disagree.[25]

Just as in considerations about the value of exercise, there is some truth in the philosophy. Overwhelming scientific evidence now confirms that the typical Western diet is too high in animal products and saturated fat, and too low in fruit, vegetables and fibre. However, there is also a high incidence of iron-deficiency anaemia in women of child-bearing age who eat a vegetarian diet containing little available iron.

If we decline God's provision for us, on the grounds that by doing so we are being kinder to animals or adopting a healthier lifestyle, we must therefore be sure that we are not rejecting God's order in creation and making idols out of the animal kingdom or our own health. Well established, traditional animal welfare societies avoid the issue of vegetarianism and work towards goals that all Christians should support, such as humane breeding establishments and abattoirs and limits to livestock transportation.

There are many more issues that could be discussed. They include the belief that cancer can be prevented by certain faddish diets (not borne out by epidemiological research), an obsession with stress and stress management, and preoccupation with various forms of meditation. In each case a valuable truth has been distorted. A balanced diet containing fruit, vitamins and minerals is beneficial to one's health, knowledge of relaxation techniques can be helpful, and in our hectic lives it can be priceless to reclaim places and times of stillness. However, when the truth is distorted, pursuit of our own happiness becomes of paramount importance and these goals become what the Bible calls idols.

There is concern in some Christian circles that several forms of CAM are vehicles for the promotion of other religious perspectives, many opposed to Christianity, and that others may even involve occult practices. Since the New Age movement believes that all spirituality is good, and that no form is better than any other, it should not surprise us if some CAM therapies have a strong spiritual influence which is very frequently not Christian in origin.

There can be a tendency for some Christians to blame the New Age for any and everything, which may be unhelpful. As stated previously, the New Age is most definitely not new, although its proponents would like us to think it is because it sounds more attractive that way. Further, by blaming the New Age movement, Christians are absolved from the responsibility to think. Provided they can label something as 'New Age', they can reject it. What will they do when the New Age disappears (as it will) and the same heresies appear under a different name? Christians need to use their minds and not be naïve.

It will probably never be possible to document with precision the more subtle spiritual hazards associated with CAM. However, it should be of concern to Christians that CAM remedies with a spiritual basis often involve the worship of other gods. As such they are clearly forbidden by God.[26] We can conclude that there will always be the need for Christians to explore whether there is a spiritual basis to a particular CAM therapy. Only after investigating this should we carefully and prayerfully consider whether to embark on such a course.

References

1. The House of Lords Select Committee on Science & Technology Sixth Report. London UK: 21 November 2000
2. Harper J. Traditional Chinese medicine for eczema. *BMJ* 1994; 308:489-490
3. www.mhra.gov.uk accessed June 2007
4. Ernst E. Adverse effects of herbal drugs in dermatology. *Br J Dermatol* 2000; 143:923-929
5. Lord G *et al.* Nephropathy caused by Chinese herbs in the UK. *Lancet* 1999; 354: 481-482
6. Renal failure associated with Chinese herbal medicines. *Current Problems in Pharmacovigilance* 1999; 25: 18
7. Jappe U *et al.* Sebotropic drug reaction resulting from kava-kava extract therapy: a new entity? *J Am Acad Dermatol* 1998; 38:104-6
8. Dasgupta A, Bernard D. Herbal remedies: effects on clinical laboratory tests. *Arch Pathol Lab Med* 2006; 130: 521-528
9. Schelosky L *et al.* Kava and dopamine antagonism. *J Neurol Neurosurg Psychiatr* 1995; 58: 639-40
10. Matthews M Jr. Association of Ginkgo biloba with intracerebral hemorrhage. *Neurology* 1998; 50: 1933-4
11. Rowin J, Lewis S. Spontaneous bilateral subdural hematomas associated with chronic Ginkgo biloba ingestion. *Neurology* 1996; 46: 1775-76
12. Gilbert G. Ginkgo biloba. [Letter]. *Neurology* 1997; 48: 1137
13. St John's Wort. *Med Letter Drugs Ther* 1997; 39: 107-8
14. Woelk H *et al.* Benefits and risks of the Hypericum extract LI 160: drug monitoring study with 3250 patients. *J Geriatr Psychiatry Neurol* 1994; 7(suppl 1): S34-38
15. Golsch S *et al.* Reversible increase in photosensitivity to UV-B caused by St John's Wort extract. *Hautartzt* 1997; 48: 240-52
16. Bove G. Acute neuropathy after exposure to sun in a patient treated with St John's Wort. [Letter] *Lancet* 1998; 352: 1121-2
17. British National Formulary, September 2007. Appendix 1 p743
18. www.medtox.org accessed July 2007
19. Fergusson A. In: *Hard Questions about Health and Healing.* London: Christian Medical Fellowship, 2005 p120-1
20. *Nucleus.* CMF, April 1994 p17-23
21. Koch K. *Occult ABC.* Grand Rapids: Kregel, 1986 p104
22. Gumprecht J. *New Age Health Care.* California USA: Promise Publishing, 1988
23. 1 Corinthians 6:19-20
24. Romans 1:25
25. Romans 14:1-4
26. Deuteronomy 5:7; Ephesians 5:11

For reflection on your own or for discussion in a small group

1. How would you classify CAM therapies?
2. How would you explain to someone that 'natural does not mean harmless'?
3. What responsibility do you think individuals should play in maintaining their own health? How can or should healthcare practitioners help with this?
4. Should the church or Christian communities be involved?

5

Fact or fiction?

Science is nothing but trained and organised common sense.

TH Huxley. *Collected Essays*

What is truth?   John 18:38

In the Introduction I outlined why we cannot afford to ignore CAM. In chapter one I showed that some treatments available on the NHS, such as psychotherapy, have not always been as thoroughly evaluated as one might expect. It is not therefore possible to define CAM as comprising all those therapeutic practices which have not been subjected to rigorous evaluation. Instead I used the definition employed by the Cochrane Collaboration, that of 'a broad domain of healing resources that encompasses all health systems, modalities, and practices and their accompanying theories and beliefs, other than those intrinsic to the politically dominant health systems of a particular society or culture in a given historical period'. In chapter two I looked briefly at the historical background to orthodox medicine and CAM. In chapter three I examined why CAM therapies have become so popular in Western societies in the least two decades. In chapter four I looked at just a few of the treatments included under the CAM umbrella and examined the potential problems associated with their unrestricted practice. In this chapter I examine how researchers, scientists and clinicians evaluate new treatments in orthodox healthcare, and how these approaches may be applied to evaluate CAM therapies.

Evaluating treatments
In order to advance the frontiers of medical knowledge, doctors and scientists can never be satisfied with existing achievements.

New treatments must continually be developed and evaluated, yet objective evaluation of new treatments is always a demanding challenge. The need for proper evaluation, possible strategies, and some of the potential problems encountered, are outlined here.

I will begin by discussing the methods which doctors and medical scientists currently use to evaluate medical (and surgical) treatments of many varieties. Historically such methods have been largely applied to orthodox medicine.

Why evaluate?

It is important that medical therapies offered to the public should be known to be effective, whether their cost is subsidised by the government or charged directly to the individual. Ineffective treatments waste the patient's time and money and may mean that the patient is denied another genuinely effective remedy. New treatments must also be shown to be safe, or at least as safe as the existing ones.

Drug development

Drug discovery arises in various ways. As discussed in chapter four, a therapeutic compound may be developed from plant sources, examples being morphine and digoxin. Sometimes good fortune, coupled with detailed observation and hard work, are responsible. An example is the discovery of penicillin by Alexander Fleming.

Alternatively, drugs may be developed rationally on the basis of existing knowledge and hypotheses about the cause of disease. Such a drug is L-dopa, used to treat Parkinson's disease. Before its development, it was known that there were reduced amounts of dopamine in the brains of patients with Parkinsonism. L-dopa is converted to dopamine following administration to the patient. The rationale for using it was therefore to restore levels of dopamine to normal.

Drug testing

Once a potential drug is discovered it undergoes extensive pharmacological testing to determine its therapeutic properties and potential side-effects. When enough is known about its safety, it is given to healthy volunteers and its effects recorded. If it is found to be safe, short-term studies are then performed on patients, followed by large scale ones often conducted over a longer period of time. Only after satisfying these stages is a new drug released onto the market. In practice only about one in 1,000 potential compounds reaches the point of testing in clinical studies, and it takes several years of research before a compound is ready for testing. Further delay occurs while the drug enters large scale clinical trials.

Throughout the world, drug regulatory authorities exist to ensure that drugs are of acceptable quality, efficacy and safety. In the UK the responsibility lies with the Health Ministers for England and Wales, Scotland and Northern Ireland, who ultimately oversee the issuing of licences and certificates for new drugs. In this way, every effort is made to ensure that only safe and effective drugs reach the public.

In 2003, the Medicines Control Agency and the Medical Devices Agency were merged to form the Medicines and Healthcare Products Regulatory Agency (MHRA). This is now the UK Department of Health's executive agency responsible for ensuring that medicines and medical devices are effective and acceptably safe. It works closely with the European Medicines Agency (EMEA), a decentralised body of the European Union with headquarters in London. The EMEA's main responsibility is the protection and promotion of public and animal health through evaluation and supervision of medicines for human and veterinary use. It has its own pharmaco-vigilance network and contributes to international activities in various ways, for example work with the European Pharmacopoeia and the World Health Organisation (WHO), and trilateral conferences on harmonisation involving the EU, Japan and the US.

Old treatments are continuously being challenged by newer ones. For doctors, deciding whether these newer treatments represent an improvement over established ones often presents the greatest challenge.

Clinical trials

Sometimes it is relatively easy to demonstrate the efficacy of a given treatment. The more predictable the outcome of the disease, and the more effective the treatment, the easier it is to prove. For example, the efficacy of penicillin in treating pneumococcal pneumonia is dramatic and easy to prove. However, striking results such as these are relatively uncommon in medicine and some kind of formal study is needed to evaluate therapies. By subjecting both orthodox medicine to more rigorous evaluation, and examining CAM therapies in this way, we will be in a better position to discover which treatments are of genuine value in fighting disease.

The placebo effect, as discussed previously, is the term given to describe the observation that one third of all people, given an inert compound to relieve a particular symptom, will report relief of that symptom. Owing to this phenomenon it is often not easy to determine whether a particular treatment is effective. Related to the placebo is the positive psychological effect of an individual investing time and money in a particular therapy. Treatment freely available in the NHS system may not be so highly valued.

There are other reasons why clinical trials are necessary, and why healthcare practitioners cannot simply rely on anecdotal reports to judge a proposed treatment's efficacy. Many conditions are self-limiting, such as the common cold or influenza in a young healthy adult. This means that they will get better in any case over time. Unless rigorous testing is used, it can be impossible to decide whether an observed improvement is due to the treatment (intervention) or to the natural history of the condition. Furthermore, many diseases are cyclical. Allergies, digestive problems such as irritable bowel syndrome, arthritis, multiple sclerosis and migraines will all fluctuate in severity and frequency of attacks. Only rigorous testing will eliminate the possibility that the intervention was given just before the condition was about to improve in any case. Finally, an intervention may be given at the end of a period of conventional treatment and may appear to be beneficial when the conventional therapy had failed. Nevertheless, it may have been that the orthodox treatment was in fact effective, but its effects took some time to become manifest. Good quality, large scale clinical trials are thus essential to help doctors evaluate new therapies more objectively.

How do we define whether a particular treatment is effective? We may state that it should be shown to alleviate one or more symptoms, or to ameliorate or cure a disease. Which symptoms we define as important will be determined both by our understanding of the natural history of the disease and by the patient's expectations. Two examples given below illustrate this.

In treating a patient with terminal cancer and a life expectancy of only a few days we may choose to give a drug which successfully relieves pain, even though we know that it could under some circumstances shorten life. In this situation the patient's quality of life becomes of greater importance than its length in days or weeks.

However, when evaluating a new treatment for heart attack we will want to examine its effect on survival after one, six or 12 months. We will probably also want to investigate its effect on the functioning of the heart muscle and the efficiency of blood flow in the coronary arteries at various times after the heart attack. In order to assess the efficacy of a given treatment in this situation we therefore first need to know what measurements will accurately predict long-term survival, as well as considering the patient's quality of life when it is prolonged.

In any one individual who receives a particular treatment the benefit of treatment should outweigh any likely hazard, or risk, associated with the treatment. Whenever doctors prescribe drugs or perform surgical procedures they have to make some assessment of the benefit to risk ratio for the individual patient.

As mentioned previously, subjective impressions of whether a particular treatment is effective are known to be potentially misleading. This is partly because doctors and patients both tend to be biased towards believing that the treatment is beneficial, and partly because of the placebo phenomenon.

A clinical trial involves the administration of one or more therapies to a group of individuals under medical supervision. There has to be some pre-existing evidence suggesting that the treatment may be beneficial, and the study should demonstrate both efficacy and any side-effects the therapy may have. It can be applied to procedures (for example a surgical operation) as well as to the administration of a drug.

At its simplest, a clinical trial may compare the efficacy and safety of two drugs, A and B. Alternatively it may compare a drug A with a placebo. The placebo is usually an inert compound with no pharmacological activity. A brief outline of some of the issues which need to be considered by doctors performing clinical trials is given below.

Numbers of patients

The study is usually carried out in a substantial number of patients. This is because all individuals are unique, and will therefore respond slightly differently to the same treatment. It is thus always potentially possible to claim that a new treatment is valuable if it has only been given to one or two patients. The number of patients required depends partly upon the expected difference in efficacy between treatments. If treatment A improves outcome by 10%, a substantial number of patients will be needed to confirm that it confers an advantage over existing treatments. If, however, treatment A is thought to improve outcome by 50%, fewer patients will be required to demonstrate the beneficial effect.

Bias

An investigator who knows which treatment a patient is receiving may in some way, even unconsciously, influence the outcome because his or her judgement is biased. In order to try and eliminate such bias in a study, clinical trials are whenever possible performed in a 'double-blind' manner. This means that neither the doctor nor the patient knows which treatment the patient is receiving until after the study is finished. Furthermore, patients are usually randomly allocated to each treatment group; hence the term 'randomised' controlled trial.

Ethics

A number of ethical issues have to be addressed in clinical trials. Examples include using uncomfortable or potentially hazardous procedures which would not normally be needed in the course of investigation or treatment, and the use of a placebo where a drug already exists which is thought to be effective.

The question of what constitutes 'informed consent' can be difficult. Where patients are asked to undergo surgery, diagnostic procedures, or take part in medical research, they are required to give what is termed 'informed consent'. The idea is that the patient should be fully aware of the nature of the procedure, and of the risks involved. In practice, most risks are extremely rare, and there will only be one or two complications which commonly arise. If one were to list all the possible risks involved in having one's appendix removed, very many patients would probably have serious doubts about the advisability of proceeding! In reality, the risks are usually extremely small. It is therefore often difficult to know how far to go in trying to explain all the details, including very remote hazards, to patients.

Clinical trials in conditions where the patients may be elderly or suffering from mental illness, or where the subjects are children, pose extra challenges. Owing to these difficulties, research institutions and hospitals conducting clinical trials must submit all research proposals to independent ethical committees, who will advise whether they consider them to be ethical. Such committees include lay members of the public as well as experienced researchers and healthcare professionals.

Given the above considerations, it is clear that clinical trials cannot be undertaken lightly and are often complex to plan and perform. In some cases several clinical trials, designed to answer the same question, produce conflicting results. This is because a large number of variables can affect the outcome of a clinical trial. These include the precise question the trial was designed to answer, the number and characteristics of the subjects studied, the dose and method of administration of the drug(s) given or the experience of the surgeon(s) involved in performing a surgical procedure, the length of treatment, the outcome measure chosen (for example death, survival at one year or the patients' perception of quality of life), the length of follow-up after cessation of treatment, and the methods used for statistical analysis.

Clinical trials are almost invariably performed in several countries with a number of different variables such as those mentioned above, and not infrequently yield apparently contradictory conclusions. Healthcare practitioners are then left in a real dilemma as to which body of evidence they can trust. In an attempt to bring together results from different clinical trials, systematic reviews have become increasingly popular. A systematic review is a summary of the medical literature that uses explicit methods to perform a thorough literature search and critical appraisal of individual studies, and uses appropriate statistical methods to combine results from studies considered to be valid. Nevertheless, not all systematic reviews are equal in their quality and thus even their interpretation is sometimes open to question.

A further limitation of classical double-blind placebo-controlled randomised trials is that they are usually conducted in highly selected patients or volunteers who may bear little resemblance to the 'average', real-life patient. Owing to understandable concerns about safety, subjects with certain medical conditions may be excluded from a study, or there may be an age cut-off above which no patients are recruited. Patients included in a study may for various reasons be more highly motivated than real-life patients to take their medication consistently and attend the hospital or surgery for regular check-ups. Even a minor adverse event may lead to the patient being withdrawn and not completing the study.

In recent years these considerations have led to increased recognition of the value of other means of evaluating effectiveness in medicine. These include so-called pragmatic randomised controlled trials, where the inclusion criteria are broader, outcomes are kept simple and normal events are allowed to influence the results, and observational studies, where a cohort of patients is studied prospectively for a defined period of time. Such studies are of course potentially highly subject to bias, but when well-conducted can nevertheless yield valuable information in a real-life setting. In particular, they recognise that individuals will not always behave in a 'textbook' fashion in response to a particular medication or intervention.

Publication

The reader should be aware that the quality of any given research is to a considerable degree judged by the journal in which it is published. Biomedical journals are ranked by their impact factor, which is a measure of how often their articles are cited in other journals. The higher the impact factor, the more prestigious the journal, and the more highly rated will be the research published in that journal. Impact factors are recalculated on an annual basis. Although controversial, impact factors do have some relevance to the general reader searching for articles on a biomedical topic, since publication of a study in a highly rated journal generally carries more weight than publication in a journal with a low impact factor.

Scientific evaluation of CAM therapies

So far we have examined ways in which doctors and clinical scientists attempt to evaluate the safety and efficacy of both new and existing treatments in an orthodox clinical setting. Many doctors believe that both the medical profession and CAM practitioners must attempt to evaluate CAM therapies using the same methods currently applied to orthodox treatments. Although the concept of evidence-based medicine is a relatively new one in CAM, a body of scientific enquiry has now emerged which merits examination.

In applying the use of clinical trials to evaluate CAM therapies, challenges arise. For instance, it is impossible to conduct a double-blind trial comparing manipulative (osteopathic or chiropractic) therapy with non-manipulative therapy. Nevertheless, as an editorial in *The Lancet* highlighted as early as 1994[1] and as we saw above, clinical studies do not necessarily have to be performed in the traditional double-blind fashion to yield valuable information.

The Lancet editorial notes, 'To carry scientific credibility, patients receiving a new treatment must be tested against a very similar control group who receive either the current standard treatment or no active treatment at all. Allocation to each group must be rigorously randomised. When the outcome is objective and completely independent of judgement by the subject or by the trialist' [for example, survival] 'blinding of either is not crucial.'

When physical treatments are being assessed, a CAM therapy can be compared with a conventional treatment (such as physiotherapy) that can be applied with equal conviction, time and attention given to each individual. More recently, the feasibility and validity of well-conducted clinical trials of CAM have been emphasised by Professor Ernst.[2] He points out that it is possible to incorporate, for example, the individualised prescribing characteristic of homoeopathy or Bach Flower Remedy proponents into clinical trials, and that several clinical trials have already provided valid information about the efficacy of CAM.

Well-designed clinical trials are a vital tool in evaluating new CAM treatments. They are essential if we are to exclude other confounding factors which may cause a CAM therapy to appear effective. Such factors include the natural history of disease (many conditions are self-limiting, that is they improve over time regardless of treatment), the placebo effect, other concurrent treatments and expectations of the practitioner or client. Trial results should be repeatable and independent of any 'magical' powers claimed by the practitioner. Such studies are crucial in furthering our understanding about whether such treatments work and if so, how they achieve their effects.

CAM therapies on trial

This section briefly considers examples of instances where controlled trials have already been performed to evaluate CAM therapies.

There is considerable evidence from randomised controlled trials of the effectiveness of spinal manipulation for back and neck pain.[3] As an illustration, a controlled North American trial conducted in Chicago examined 178 patients with back pain who were randomly assigned to receive osteopathic manual therapy or standard medical therapy.[4] Patients in both groups improved over 12 weeks and there was no statistically significant difference between them in any of the primary outcome measures. However, those receiving osteopathic treatment required significantly less medication (painkillers, anti-inflammatory agents and muscle relaxants) than the patients receiving standard care.

Professor Ernst has reviewed 17 systematic reviews of controlled trials of homoeopathy.[5] He concluded that these studies fail to provide strong evidence in favour of homoeopathy, and that no homoeopathic remedy has been proven to yield clinical effects that differ from placebo.

Several studies have evaluated the use of acupuncture in the UK, Europe, US and China. It has been hypothesised that release of the body's own (endogenous) pain-relieving chemicals (endorphins or opioids) is increased following acupuncture and that this may contribute to pain relief.[6] Some investigators have recorded objective physiological effects during acupuncture resulting in diminished awareness of pain (termed an increased pain threshold). A degree of caution is required in interpreting these findings, since pain relief associated with placebos is also thought to be mediated by endogenous opioids and can be blocked by naloxone, an inhibitor of the actions of morphine. However, to quote the *BMJ* editorial referenced above, acupuncture does appear to have 'some physiological respectability'.

Despite these findings, a systematic review of randomised controlled trials of acupuncture for neck pain did not support the hypothesis that acupuncture is an effective treatment for this condition.[7] A review of controlled trials of acupuncture for various gynaecological conditions concluded that doubt remains about the effectiveness of acupuncture in such circumstances.[8] The author considered acupuncture and acupressure promising for dysmenorrhoea, and acupuncture for infertility, but stressed that further studies are required. However, a systematic review of randomised controlled trials of acupuncture for recurrent headaches failed to provide evidence for any effect of acupuncture in headache.[9]

In the last decade there has been a number of controlled clinical trials conducted to evaluate the efficacy of herbal remedies, as illustrated by the following three examples. Glucosamine is a naturally-occurring substance found in cartilage and produced synthetically for the food supplements market. It has similar actions to chondroitin, which is found in bovine tracheal cartilage, has anti-inflammatory activity and is thought to rebuild cartilage. Glucosamine has become a popular 'natural' treatment for osteoarthritis; several randomised controlled trials have been conducted and most have yielded positive results. A systematic review in 2000 included 15 trials of glucosamine and chondroitin and was cautiously optimistic, although the authors reported a numbers of weaknesses in methods used and a possible degree of publication bias.[10] In a separate, older study comparing glucosamine with ibuprofen, the clinical outcome was similar in both groups but more adverse effects were recorded with ibuprofen.[11]

Cranberry bushes are evergreen shrubs native to temperate regions of the US, and cranberry juice has been advocated as a remedy for urinary tract infections since 1840 when German scientists proposed that it had antibacterial activity. The mechanism of action is unclear although it has been suggested that cranberry juice prevents bacteria from sticking to the inner walls of the urinary tract. There is evidence that drinking 300ml of cranberry juice daily for six months reduces the risk of urinary tract infections when compared with a placebo.[12] A Cochrane Review in 2000 examined four randomised controlled trials, of which three were in favour of cranberry juice.[13] However, owing to the poor quality of these studies, the authors questioned the reliability of the findings.

Saw palmetto is a dwarf palm native to coastal regions of southern states in North America, particularly Florida and South Carolina, and an extract was traditionally used by local populations to treat bladder or urethral irritation. A systematic review of 18 randomised controlled trials examining saw palmetto in the treatment of benign prostatic hypertrophy concluded that it significantly improves symptoms and flow measures compared with placebo.[14] When compared with a conventional agent, finasteride, it appears to have similar efficacy with fewer adverse effects, but no long term data are available.

Regulation of CAM - therapists and therapies

In addition to close scrutiny of CAM therapies by well-designed clinical studies, regulation of CAM practitioners is necessary. Such regulation should include four elements.

1. *Registration*
   There should be a register of all CAM practitioners. It should be open to public scrutiny and entry to the register should be limited to competent practitioners.

2. *Code of Conduct*
   There should be guidelines regarding the professional standards required, competence to practise, and ethical conduct.

3. *Core Curriculum*
   There should be a formal training structure with a core curriculum.

4. *Basic Medical Science Training*
   Training in the basic medical sciences should be compulsory. CAM practitioners should be aware of the limits of their

competence and should be taught to diagnose conditions which are contraindications to the treatment they offer.

As a result of such measures, osteopathic practitioners should for example be able to recognise signs suggestive of a bone tumour and a massage therapist should be able to recognise features suggesting deep vein thrombosis. Neither cancer nor deep vein thrombosis will respond to CAM therapy, and either condition is likely to worsen, with serious consequences, if not treated by conventional methods. There should be clear protocols for communicating with medical practitioners, and CAM therapists should be prevented from revoking prescriptions given by a doctor. Last but not least, good quality research and continuing professional development should be encouraged.

An example of how regulation of CAM therapies has progressed over the last decade is provided by the traditional herbal registration scheme. As previously noted, most herbal medicines on the UK market are currently unlicensed, and standards vary greatly. Under the 2004 European Directive on traditional herbal medicinal products, all manufactured traditional herbal medicines placed on the market will have to meet the requirements of the Directive. Products will be required to meet assured standards of quality, safety and patient information; minor health claims are allowed on the basis of evidence of traditional use. In order to register a product, companies have to submit a dossier to the MHRA demonstrating that it meets the requirements of the scheme. There is transitional protection until 2011 for products that were legally on the UK market before April 2004, and the MHRA expects a progressive increase in the number of products registered as 2011 approaches. Products with a Traditional Herbal Registration have a 'THR' number on the label; licensed medicines have a PL (Product Licence) number.

In November 2006 the MHRA granted the first UK product registration under the European Directive on traditional herbal medicinal products. This was given to Bioforce (UK) Ltd for Atrogel Arnica Gel, an arnica gel traditionally used for symptomatic relief of muscular aches and pains, stiffness, sprains, bruises and swelling after contusions.

Two months earlier, in September 2006, the MHRA introduced a new scheme, the National Rules Scheme, to improve and strengthen regulation of homoeopathic products in the UK. This followed a public consultation in 2005. Companies are encouraged to register new homoeopathic medicines under the scheme, with the option of re-registering certain existing products. Companies are allowed to include information about the treatment and relief of minor, self-limiting conditions (for example common colds, cough, hay fever or chilblains) based on the use of the product within the homoeopathic tradition. All homoeopathic remedies authorised under this scheme have clear and comprehensive patient information leaflets, with the goal of helping consumers use their medicines safely and effectively. Products authorised under the National Rules Scheme have to comply with recognised standards of quality, safety and patient information. Finally, all homoeopathic medicines now fall within the scope of the Yellow Card Scheme, which allows patients and healthcare professionals to reported suspected side effects to the MHRA.

While the goal of ensuring that all herbal and homoeopathic remedies meet certain safety and quality standards is obviously very welcome, it does not guarantee the efficacy of these products. It may indeed confer an appearance of respectability to such products not borne out by scientific evidence. Registration will certainly help to ensure that these remedies will not cause harm. However, registration alone is obviously not sufficient to guarantee that a given remedy is beneficial and there remains a need for good quality clinical trials to establish or disprove the efficacy of such treatments.

Conclusions

In this chapter I have illustrated ways in which conventional methods could be applied more widely to evaluate and regulate certain CAM therapies. In chapter six I will examine some practical ways in which individual Christians might evaluate such therapies from a more personal perspective. I will also consider what specific responses Christian doctors might make to the challenges posed by CAM.

References

1. Editorial, *The Lancet* 1994; 343:553-554
2. Ernst E. Complementary medicine: clinical trials. *Pharm J* 2005; 275:612
3. Vickers A, Zollmann C. ABC of complementary medicine: the manipulative therapies - osteopathy and chiropractic. *BMJ* 1999; 319: 1176-1179
4. Andersson G *et al.* A comparison of osteopathic spinal manipulation with standard care for patients with low back pain. *New Engl J Med* 1999; 341: 1426-1431
5. Ernst E. A systematic review of systematic reviews of homoeopathy. *Br J Clin Pharm* 2002; 54: 577-582
6. How does acupuncture work? *BMJ* (Clinical Research Editorial) 1981; 283: 746-748
7. White A, Ernst E. A systematic review of randomized controlled trials of acupuncture for neck pain. *Rheumatology* 1999; 38: 143-147
8. White A. A review of controlled trials of acupuncture for women's reproductive health care. *J Fam Plann Reprod Health Care* 2003; 29: 233-36
9. Melchart D *et al.* Acupuncture for idiopathic headache. *The Cochrane Library.* Update Software, 2000
10. McAllindon T *et al.* Glucosamine and chondroitin for treatment of osteoarthritis. A systematic quality assessment and meta-analysis. *JAMA* 2000; 283: 1469-75
11. Miller-Fabbender H *et al.* Glucosamine sulphate compared to ibuprofen in osteoarthritis of the knee. *Osteoarthr Cartilage* 1994; 2: 61-69
12. Avorn J *et al.* Reduction of bacteriuria and pyuria after ingestion of cranberry juice. *JAMA* 1994; 272: 590
13. Jepson R *et al.* Cranberries for preventing urinary tract infections. *The Cochrane Library.* Update Software, 2000
14. Wilt T *et al.* Saw palmetto extracts for treatment of benign prostatic hyperplasia. *JAMA* 1998; 280: 1604-9

For reflection on your own or for discussion in a small group

1. Why are clinical trials important in evaluating new treatments?
2. What questions should you ask about a particular piece of research in order to try and judge its quality?
3. Why is regulation of medicines and healthcare practitioners important?
4. Does regulation of CAM ensure efficacy of CAM therapies?

6

A Christian response

Beware that you do not lose the substance by grasping at the shadow.

Aesop's Fables: 'The Dog and The Shadow'

Test everything. Hold on to the good.

I Thessalonians 5:21

Medicine and the Bible

Before discussing how we might respond to CAM therapies I want to consider briefly what the Bible has to say about medicine. Despite many references in the Bible to sin, sickness, health and healing, there are few direct references to medical practice.

Much of the Old Testament describes the history of the Jewish nation. During Joseph's life his family, seventy people in all, settled in Egypt. Later, under a new ruler (Pharaoh), their descendants, the Israelites, were forced into slavery. Alarmed by the continued expansion of these foreigners in his country, the Pharaoh ordered that the midwives should kill all baby boys born into Jewish families. Two midwives who disobeyed his command were commended and blessed by God.[1] This account endorses the view that all life is precious in God's eyes and that infanticide is immoral. It also makes it clear that God's people relied on the midwives and medical practitioners of their day just as their neighbours did.

There is a brief reference to the part our mental state can play in our physical health in the book of Proverbs,[2] where it states that a 'cheerful heart is good medicine'. No-one is likely to disagree with this commonsense approach.

The Apocrypha is a collection of writings considered to contain teaching which is edifying for the church but which lacks the divine authority of the rest of Scripture. Ecclesiasticus is a collection of writings giving practical advice for life. In this book, medical skill is seen as God's gift.[3] 'Honour the physician with the honour due to him, according to your need of him, for the Lord created him; for healing comes from the Most High... The Lord created medicines from the earth, and a sensible man will not despise them... he gave skill to men that he might be glorified in his marvellous works. By them he heals and takes away pain...'

The writer of the third Gospel, Luke, was a doctor by profession.[4] As one might expect, he sometimes includes medical details omitted in the other gospels. In his account he records Jesus healing a woman with persistent haemorrhage.[5] He says with sober realism, 'And a woman was there who had been subject to bleeding for twelve years, but no-one could heal her'. Doctors failed in those days just as they do now, but Jesus was able to heal her.

What can we learn from these references? Firstly, that only God has the power to give or withhold healing. All healing should therefore be regarded as being ultimately divine in origin. Secondly, in his compassion, God has entrusted medical knowledge and skills as a gift to mankind. Consequently he expects his people to consult doctors. Thirdly, it is recognised that there will always be conditions which doctors are unable to cure.

In practice, I believe these considerations mean several things. Christians should be careful not to reject medicine or its practitioners just because they do not always share their beliefs. Faith in God is not required to exercise these skills, and many brilliant and compassionate doctors have been, are, and always will be, atheists or agnostics.

Christians can help those who have fallen into the trap of thinking that conventional medicine will always be successful. Doctors fail, treatments fail, and patients remain ill or die. As we have seen, many today expect instant and complete cures, and so are disappointed. Christians have the opportunity to point them to an all-powerful, all-loving God, but they must remember that God's omnipotence and benevolence do not guarantee us physical or psychological health in this life. When he does not heal, his love and presence remain with us to support us.

Christian objectivity about CAM

There is evidently a need for objectivity about orthodox medicine. What about CAM therapies? There are four general questions we can ask about any new therapy being offered, outlined below.

Facts

Do the claims for this therapy fit the facts? Some answers to this question are not as difficult for a layperson to find as one might think.

In some cases publicity is obviously misleading. It does not require medical qualifications to spot this type of publicity once made aware of it. While not necessarily associated with occult practices, such publicity is blatantly untruthful. Examples are claims that one form of treatment will cure a vast number of diseases. Such publicity comes in leaflets distributed in a variety of ways.

One such flyer I received, unsolicited and pinned to my windscreen, reads as follows: 'This is a guide to a much wider range of ailments which can be treated …**Pains of all kinds:** arthritis, sciatica, tennis elbow, back pain, tendenitis [misspelt], headache, trigeminal neuralgia, lumbago. **Disorders:** Infections – bronchitis, cold, flu, Ear nose and throat – hay fever, sinusitis, tinitus [misspelt], Alimentary – duodenal ulcer, indigestion, gastric ulcers, obesity, haemorrhoids, Circulatory – anaemia, palpitations, high/low blood pressure, Pulmonary – bronchiectasis, Dermatological – acne, psoriasis, eczema, herpes, Genito-Urinary & Reproductive – dysmenorrhoea, menopausal symptoms, impotence, menstrual disorder, cystitis, Endoctrinal [misspelt] – hormonal problem, adrenal insufficiency, Mental-Emotional – anxiety, insomnia, depression, peripheral neuritis, stress, Other Problems – smoking, weight, alcoholism'.

Not only is this list ridiculously extensive, it is also a quite random selection of disorders, some of which overlap. In reality, one drug is never the solution for all diseases, although it may indeed have several applications.

Scientific basis

It is important to establish whether there is any scientific basis for the therapy on offer. The practitioner offering treatment should be able and willing to provide this kind of information. If they are not, it should alert us to the possibility that either they themselves are not competent or else that the treatment has no scientific basis. If it has no scientific basis, we must bear in mind that it may not be harmless. As I have illustrated previously, even apparently innocuous substances may have harmful physical side-effects. Alternatively it may be based on a psychic form of healing. If we are in doubt regarding the validity of scientific claims, we should be able to consult our general practitioner or specialist about the treatment.

The therapist's worldview

As we have explored previously, behind a number of CAM therapies on offer today, although certainly not all of them, there lies a hidden, spiritual agenda. How do we recognise this and how should we respond?

Christians are clearly warned in the Bible to avoid involvement in the occult. This implies that they should be careful to avoid treatments associated with occult practices. By occult practices I mean practices characterised by mystical or supernatural phenomena. God makes it very clear in the Old Testament that his people are to have no dealings whatsoever with spiritualists or mediums of any kind.[6] However, sometimes one therapy can be offered by two different practitioners with wholly opposing views and beliefs. Consider the case of acupuncture, which illustrates this very clearly. Several articles have been written by evangelical Christians denouncing acupuncture as a work of the devil to be avoided at all costs. A number of equally evangelical Christians have studied acupuncture in some depth and have come to opposite conclusions.

Why is there such a difference of opinion? The former Christians have denounced acupuncture on the basis that it is connected with the occult. However, the word occult can also be used to describe phenomena beyond ordinary human understanding, or not at present explicable in Western scientific terms. This is not the meaning given in the Bible[7] where it is associated with evil spirits and divination, which are clearly condemned.

The practice and theory of acupuncture date back to at least 540 BC in China. The theory put forward to explain the basis of acupuncture was as follows. As mentioned in chapter two, life was thought to be dependent on a combination in specific proportions of yang (energy from the sun) and yin (energy from the earth). Sickness was attributed to an imbalance of these two energies.

Health was thought to be maintained by movement of the vital breath in channels between the various vital organs. These channels were thought to run in lines up and down the body, named after the organ they served and often depicted on models as lines or meridians. The models served merely as anatomy models to demonstrate the various lines and anatomy points. It was thought that it was possible to influence the movement of this vital force and restore the normal flow by stimulating these channels with needles at certain points along their course.

A traditional acupuncturist will work on this basis and may well also prescribe herbal medicine and give advice about diet. A modern acupuncturist, often a Western doctor, will take a straightforward history, formulate a diagnosis in traditional Western medical terms, may not believe in the existence of meridians, and may find his own acupuncture points. Fine disposable injection needles are as effective as traditional acupuncture needles.

The traditional Chinese view of health and disease differs from our own. However, there is no association between acupuncture in traditional Chinese medicine and seeking help from outside spiritual forces, consulting astrological charts or signs, or any type of fortune telling.

The controversy has probably arisen because in some cases Christians have failed to realise that a people's basic philosophy of life will determine that people's interpretation of events in all areas of life, regardless of whether their experiences are good, bad or neutral in themselves. Any phenomena in a society, whether earthquakes, diseases, famines or droughts, are open to spiritual explanation. The phenomenon of acupuncture was discovered in a non-Christian culture and interpreted in a non-Christian framework.

We can reject the traditional interpretation of acupuncture because we now have some knowledge of how it may work in physiological terms, but this does not mean that we have to reject acupuncture itself.

In reality, the concept of health being a balance of opposing forces is not unusual or particularly non-Christian. The Greeks proposed that illness resulted from an imbalance of four basic humours or fluids (bile, phlegm, blood and black bile or melancholy), and this theory was held to be valid until the mid-19th century. As we saw in chapter three, the concept of imbalance in a finely tuned system may in fact be valid. Autonomic nervous function is considered to be maintained by a balance between opposing sympathetic and parasympathetic systems. Muscle groups are categorised into opposing groups, hormones are described as having opposite and thus balancing actions, and there is considered to be a critical acid-base balance in the body.

What is obviously contrary to Christian belief is the Chinese philosophy that the source of all life is the Tao ('the way'), that the whole cosmos is interrelated, and that man remains healthy by attuning himself to the balance of the cosmos. We can and should reject this philosophy, but we should bear in mind that all events, including the year's seasons, work and marriage were seen within this philosophy. Just as we do not reject the concepts of seasons, work and marriage because we reject this ancient non-Christian philosophy, we do not on this basis have to reject acupuncture.

Consider two modern-day acupuncturists. The first may be a consultant anaesthetist in a busy district general hospital, trying to give a patient with severe, unremitting pain some short-term relief. The second may be a spiritualist, or 'healer' whose treatment is only part of a programme involving the frankly occult. Christians need to be discerning enough to distinguish between these two types of treatment on offer. The above example is obviously clear-cut; others will in real life be less so. If in doubt, a few simple questions asked of the practitioner should quickly reveal his or her viewpoint.

As we saw in chapter five, there is some evidence that acupuncture may be beneficial in certain circumstances. In such situations I think it should be received as part of the broad spectrum of God's gifts. Where there is a spiritual association it should be rejected.

Motives
The therapist

Christians believe in the existence of evil and consequently in the existence of sin. Trying to live in this world with the consequences of our own sin, and the sin of others, is a challenge facing Christians and non-Christians alike. No-one would pretend that it is ever possible to have absolutely pure motives for one's actions. Indeed, even impure motives can be harnessed for good. Desire for money or prestige can drive someone to the heights of their chosen career and service to others. Nevertheless, I think that there are some principles that can be set out when examining motives behind CAM therapies.

An overwhelming desire for money, prestige or power may lie behind the more dubious practices now offered. There is obviously nothing inherently wrong in a practitioner charging a reasonable fee for private services, but if the fee seems excessive, we should perhaps consider again the real motive behind this so-called treatment. It has been suggested that the success of some CAM therapists results from money changing hands. If we have invested hard-earned cash in a course of treatment, and with it a little bit of ego, we may be more likely to view the results in a positive light in order to justify the expense. When genuinely effective and safe treatments are being offered by CAM practitioners, money will not be their prime concern, but rather the well-being of their patients.

In exactly the same way, the greater the desire for publicity, fame or power, the more likely it is that the treatment on offer is doubtful in its safety or efficacy. An example of a case where desire for fame and money was apparently of greater importance than the safety or efficacy of the treatment was reviewed in 1993.[8] This doctor practised medicine for only two years after qualifying. Nine years later he opened an allergy clinic. In 1993 he was found guilty by the General Medical Council of touting for patients using a publicity agent, and of injecting a patient with a substance he knew would harm him.

Warning bells could probably have sounded earlier. He had previously been featured in many newspaper articles, highlights of which included: 'Allergy plight of a nice girl Nicky – one sip of vodka turns me into a sex maniac' (*News of the World* magazine) and 'Women could be turned on by a chunk of cheddar' (*People*).[9] This is probably not the kind of publicity patients would either expect or wish for their physician.

Furthermore, a letter to his publicity agent reads: 'Herewith the letter from Mrs Massey. I think you will agree it's got the beginnings of a nice story. To re-emphasise, I would like this one played a little bit special if you can. Try to get it as a "Dr [X] does it again", not just a patient story. The effect from the *Sunday Express* article is just beginning to wane slightly and a boost now would be absolutely terrific and see us right through to Christmas.' It only takes commonsense to see that the motive behind this man's practice was not just the well-being of his patients. Furthermore, the techniques of 'clinical ecology' which he used have not been scientifically validated.

The General Medical Council (GMC), which regulates doctors' professional conduct in the UK, does not prohibit advertising but does provide guidance. Their current recommendations (contained in their 2006 *Good Medical Practice* document) on providing and publishing information about medical services include making sure that the information is both factual and verifiable. They also advise that medical practitioners must not 'make unjustifiable claims about the quality or outcomes of ...services' in information provided to patients. Information 'must not offer guarantees of cures, nor exploit patients' vulnerability or lack of medical knowledge'. Furthermore, doctors 'must not put pressure on people to use a service, for example by arousing ill-founded fears for their future health'.[10]

The Patient

We have seen that conventional medicine often fails to bring a cure or even relief for a large number of patients suffering from a variety of diseases. It is vital that research should continue to pursue new avenues of treatment.

However, it is the view of some Christians in the more extreme charismatic sections of the church that, because sickness results from sin in the world, and because God is all-powerful and all-loving, it is never God's will for us to be ill. Failure to be healed is therefore attributed to sin or unbelief on the part of the patient.

I have seen the appalling devastation this teaching can bring to patients already suffering from dreadful diseases. I have heard the anguish of teenagers and university students facing premature death from the inherited disease cystic fibrosis when they are exposed to this cruel lie. David Watson recounted his distress associated with facing a similar situation when dying of bowel cancer.[11] He had at least the benefit of being older, wiser, and nearer the natural end of his life. Christian leaders must exercise responsibility, sensitivity and caution in these areas. Otherwise they may be guilty of destroying the faith of children and other vulnerable people.

What does the Bible say about this issue of healing? We have seen that the Bible is clear that God can always heal, in whatever way he chooses. However, there is no guarantee that in this life he always will heal. Jesus' followers were not always able to heal the sick.[12] Paul had to leave his friend Trophimus unwell at Miletus[13] and was apparently unable to heal his colleague Epaphroditus, even though the latter nearly died of his illness.[14] Paul advised Timothy to use a little wine as a medicine when suffering from 'frequent illnesses'.[15] Paul himself suffered from illness,[16] and his reference to a thorn in the flesh which God did not remove[17] has entered widespread use in colloquial English language.

Michael Green makes the point that it should not surprise us if God does not always heal us physically. He says, 'How people would rush to Christianity (and for all the wrong motives) if it carried with it automatic exemption from sickness! What a nonsense it would make of Christian virtues like longsuffering, patience and endurance… What a wrong impression it would give of salvation if physical wholeness were perfectly realised on earth whilst spiritual wholeness were partly reserved for heaven! What a very curious thing it would be if God were to decree death for all his children whilst not allowing illness for any of them!'[18]

We do not know why God allows suffering in this world. No-one should pretend to have all the answers. What Christians hold onto is that Jesus Christ, by allowing himself to be crucified, took part in our physical and spiritual anguish. We are thus never alone in our suffering. Perhaps the church needs to re-develop a theology of suffering, without denying the wonderful deeds that God can and does perform in the 21st century.

As Christians we may therefore need to examine our own motives when seeking CAM therapies. Is our highest priority to honour God? Or have we fallen into that familiar trap of believing lies about God? We should always pray as we seek conventional treatment. The church also has a role to play. If God does not heal us, and our suffering becomes unbearable, we may need to remember that Jesus knows the reality of excruciating physical pain.

A Christian response to CAM

There are a number of areas where Christians, both healthcare professionals and members of the public, can play an active role in responding positively to the challenge presented by CAM therapies. These largely have to do with the reasons for the rise in its popularity, which we discussed in chapter three. I explore some possible approaches.

Greater expectations

Healthcare practitioners need to be responsible in giving realistic expectations to patients. This may be as a general practitioner, specialist nurse, hospital clinician or in public broadcasting. Our enthusiasm for a particular new treatment must always be tempered with realism.

Greater disappointment

Healthcare practitioners must be honest about the prognosis in chronic disease. Obviously this does not mean doctors or nurses always have to tell their patient unwelcome news that he or she does not want to hear, but they should encourage their patients to ask questions. We can all learn from the communication skills developed within the hospice movement, and we should never think that we have 'arrived' in this challenging area. Healthcare practitioners need to recognise that many patients want to be empowered to live as well as they possibly can with their condition. CAM therapists are ahead of conventional practitioners in this respect and we could certainly learn from their approaches. This may include educating patients to invest in their own health and sense of well-being, as well as helping them to realise that a 'quick fix' mechanistic approach is rarely if ever available as a solution for chronic illness. Arthur Kleinman, Professor of Medical Anthropology and Psychiatry at Harvard Medical School, has written extensively on chronic illness, emphasising the impact of cultural and social values on patients' perception of their condition, and the vital role in healing of the wider dimensions, psychological and spiritual, of the doctor-patient relationship.[19]

Doctors should be honest about possible side-effects of a planned treatment. It may not be appropriate to detail all the fine print, but frequent or serious complications should be discussed. Again, encouraging the patient to ask questions should enable any overriding concerns they may have to be declared openly. When considering publicity and patient information for research studies, clinics or services, doctors should follow the GMC recommendations outlined above.

As professionals, doctors and nurses need to look again at the support we give, or fail to give, to our patients. We need imaginative ways of saving time and delegating clerical and technical tasks, and we may need to press for recruitment of non-medical staff to broaden the emotional support available for patients.

Supporting the healthcare team

Consultants and general practitioners should examine constructive ways in which the working patterns of junior doctors can be made compatible with quality of life. It has been said that on some occasions junior doctors lack compassion because they work in a system which affords them no compassion. In the past this may not have been surprising when many of their tasks were performed at times when they could not safely drive a car or fly a plane. Although shift patterns of working have now been introduced to limit the length of working hours, these arrangements can nevertheless have detrimental effects on family life and friendships. Likewise, those in the nursing and allied healthcare professions are frequently under pressure, working overtime to cover sickness or staffing cuts and receiving little recognition, financial or otherwise, for their efforts. Senior healthcare professionals need to be alert to these pressures, and provide practical support wherever possible.

If doctors are to continue to provide a professional service to patients, consultants and general practitioners need to retain some authority within the NHS. They will have to insist on having adequate numbers of qualified staff to perform the various tasks required. This will require prayer, imagination and wisdom.

Harnessing new resources
Building design

We saw in chapter two that environmental factors outside clinical practice can affect individual health, and in chapter three we noted Florence Nightingale's comments on how the hospital setting can influence patients' recovery from illness. There is now growing evidence that the design of hospital buildings can modify the length of inpatient stay, and patients' perceptions of the quality of healthcare staff and the treatments they receive.[20] I suspect that the physical hospital or primary care environment also has a hitherto neglected effect on the attitudes and well-being of healthcare practitioners themselves.

Christians with roles in commissioning new hospital or primary care buildings and facilities, and those with responsibility for their execution, such as architects, must acquaint themselves with current research in this area. They may thus contribute very significantly to improving public health. Members of the public in a local area may also influence this process effectively by contributing imaginatively in the planning stages. Maggie's Centres, the first of which was opened in Edinburgh in 1996, offer an example of what the private and charitable sector can achieve. Maggie's Centres aim to provide information, emotional support and relaxation and stress management for patients with cancer 'within a thoughtfully designed environment that conveys respect and support for the individual'.[21] They employ well known architects with a mission statement to 'make space which makes people feel better'.

The Medical Humanities

Community arts projects have been shown to enable those with mental health problems to grow in confidence and independence and to play a more active role in community life.[22] Art therapists, church groups and local council members may be able to promote development of similar successful projects.

Interest in using the arts, including poetry and music, in caring for patients and in the education of healthcare practitioners, is also growing.[23] Dr Rita Charon, a practising internist at Columbia University Medical Center, has a doctorate in literary studies and has pioneered the clinical practice of narrative medicine. Critical of a purely biological reductionist approach to illness, her view is that the 'revolving sets of specialists' and 21st century technology fail to allow patients to find meaning in their illness, and she believes that the study of literature can help improve doctors' listening skills and capacity for empathy.[24] Some orthodox doctors may be dismissive of such methods but Christians should surely be ready to evaluate these approaches, recognising God's role as Creator and the ultimate source of all human creativity. It has been observed that, 'unlike science, which is concerned with the general, the repeatable elements in nature, medicine, *albeit using science* [italics mine], is concerned with the uniqueness of individual patients. In its concern for the particular and the unique, medicine resembles the arts.'[25]

The role of community

In chapter three we noted that the rise in single households has led to an increased, unmet need for human contact and a listening ear. Secular writers are recognising the contribution of a materialistic focus in society to the epidemic of depression currently affecting Western nations.[26] Bruce Levine, a North American clinical psychologist, proposes as a solution living in community and modelling face-to-face emotional and economic interdependence.[27] He also highlights the value of social activism in promoting meaningful relationships and improving well-being. The New Testament believers modelled vibrant community living, and social activism is at the heart of many radical and reforming Christian movements. Within the church we have a tailor-made resource at our finger tips, if only we can treasure it and help it bear fruit.

Research and education

As Christian healthcare practitioners we must attempt to model integrated, compassionate healthcare for our students. Furthermore, we must never lose sight of the fact that the interests of future patients will be served by cutting-edge medical research. This may include delivering high quality, motivational tuition to students, attracting dedicated graduates and publicising the need for adequate funding.

Society

Christian healthcare workers need to be sensitive to the special needs of ethnic minorities. We may need to employ more interpreters or set up special clinics where their interests are better met. We need to consider whether we are contributing to racial prejudice and possibly misogyny within the medical profession. Ethnic minorities and women need greater representation in senior healthcare positions. Inequalities in healthcare provision and accessibility should be recognised and dealt with so far as we are able. For some of us this will mean dealing with personal prejudices, for others it may mean political involvement.

We need to reform paternalistic attitudes towards patients and defensiveness in the face of effective CAM therapies. The contempt in which the orthodox medical profession has held osteopaths for many years is an obvious example. Christian doctors should support, and not despise, patients who want to know more about CAM therapies, particularly since such interest may reflect, at least in part, their disappointment with orthodox medicine. Healthcare workers should however be prepared to point out spiritual dangers as well as physical ones.

Finally, there appears to be a section of the medical profession which, only too aware of the faults of previous generations of doctors, is trying to make amends by welcoming CAM remedies uncritically. This has its own dangers. If Christian doctors will repent of past mistakes and then seek wisdom from God, he will surely help us exercise discernment.

What about prayer?
I have already alluded to the physical and psychological healing that God can bring to individuals in response to prayer in the context of the Christian church. Such healing may obviously occur independently of medical treatment, but it tends to be sporadic. It may be confirmed by medical experts. Christians are urged to pray,[28] and as doctors we should clearly support this teaching. If we are unsure how to proceed, Andrew Fergusson has provided a valuable guide for Christians as to how to pray for healing.[29]

Yet the power of prayer cannot be reproduced or compared with conventional drugs in large clinical trials. I believe this will remain one of the paradoxes facing Christian doctors until the end of time. I do not believe there are any easy answers because, in the end, none of us can dictate to God. Jesus the Great Physician is also 'the Lion of the tribe of Judah'.[30]

Conclusion
It is unrealistic to expect that Christians will ever agree on all aspects of CAM. Within the church they disagree all too openly on aspects

such as the role of women, the origins and implications of homosexuality, and the role of the church in politics. My own views, outlined in this chapter, will doubtless not be accepted by all. It is part of the glory of God's creation that he made us all very different and that we do not respond to him like robots. Having accepted the authority of the Bible, and the absolute truths it contains, we have to decide for ourselves what is right. Let us in humility consult the Bible, pray, think, and act, preferably with others. When we feel daunted we should recall God's promise that 'Never will I leave you; never will I forsake you'.[31]

References

1. Exodus 1:15-22
2. Proverbs 17:22
3. Ecclesiasticus 38:1-15
4. Colossians 4:14
5. Luke 8:43-48
6. Leviticus 20:27
7. Deuteronomy 18:9-14 and Isaiah 47:13-15
8. Kay A. Alternative allergy and the General Medical Council. *BMJ* 1993; 306:122-124
9. Wood B. Keep taking the tabloids. *New Statesman Society* 1992; 31 July p14-15
10. www.gmc-uk.org/guidance accessed November 2007
11. Watson D. *Fear No Evil.* UK: Hodder & Stoughton, reprinted 1994
12. Luke 9:38-40
13. 2 Timothy 4:20
14. Philippians 2:25-27
15. 1 Timothy 5:23
16. Galatians 4:13-15
17. 2 Corinthians 12:7-9
18. Green M. *I Believe in the Holy Spirit.* UK: Hodder & Stoughton, 1985
19. Kleinman A. *The illness narratives: suffering, healing, and the human condition.* USA: Basic Books, 1989
20. Wells-Thorpe J. In: *The Healing Environment*, eds Kirklin D, Richardson R. London UK: Royal College of Physicians, 2003 p11-23
21. www.maggiescentres.org accessed November 2007
22. Anderson M. In: *The Healing Environment*, eds Kirklin D, Richardson R. London UK: Royal College of Physicians, 2003 p101-123
23. Kirklin D, Richardson R, eds. *Medical Humanities: a Practical Introduction.* London UK: Royal College of Physicians: 2001
24. Charon R. *Narrative Medicine.* New York: Oxford University Press, 2006
25. Calman K, Downie R. Why arts courses for medical curricula? *Lancet* 1996; 347:1499-1500
26. www.brucelevine.net accessed November 2007
27. Levine B. Mass society and mass depression. *Ecologist*; October 2007 p48-51
28. James 5:14
29. Fergusson A. How should Christians pray for healing? In: *Hard Questions about Health and Healing.* London UK: CMF, 2005 p133-143
30. Revelation 5:5
31. Hebrews 13:5

For reflection on your own or for discussion in a small group

1. Do you think God always heals his people of illness in this life? If not, why?
2. How can prayer be integrated into holistic care?
3. If you are a healthcare practitioner, how can you help to restore public trust in your profession?
4. If, instead, you are a member of the public, what qualities do you value most in a doctor or nurse? Do you take the trouble to give positive feedback when it is due, or do you only comment when you have a complaint?
5. How can you or your church contribute to your local community in a way which benefits residents?

7

The essential A to Z guide

On each side of the river stood the tree of life, bearing twelve crops of fruit, yielding its fruit every month. And the leaves of the tree are for the healing of the nations. Revelation 22:2

I love fruit, when it is expensive. Sir Arthur Pinero. *Second Mrs Tanqueray, I*

The following guide gives a brief overview of a selection of the most commonly encountered CAM therapies. In each case the origin and rationale for the therapy are outlined, as are current evidence for its efficacy, major contraindications and/or potential side-effects. Owing to space constraints in a book of this size the list is not exhaustive, neither is the information complete. For further details the reader is strongly recommended to consult the references given at the end of the chapter.

Acupuncture

Originating in China and traditionally a branch of Chinese medicine, acupuncture was well developed by the 1st century BC. The underlying concept is that of *qi*, or *chi*, an invisible life energy force which is thought to travel through the body along defined pathways called meridians. Over 350 acupuncture points have been defined on these meridians. Needles are inserted into the body just below the skin at these points in the belief that the body is thereby stimulated to correct its energy flow and balance, resulting in restoration of health.

No evidence has been found for the existence of *qi* or the meridians. However, Western practitioners have sought a rational explanation of the effects of acupuncture by suggesting that acupuncture sites allow nerves to be stimulated. Acupuncture has been shown to release naturally occurring opioid peptides, or endorphins, which are also released during childbirth and vigorous exercise, and which reduce pain. Serotonin, another chemical messenger implicated in enhancing mood, can also be released. This has led some modern acupuncturists to refine the technique using electrical stimulation of acupuncture needles (electro-acupuncture). Low frequency (2-4Hz) high intensity electrical stimulation is used to stimulate release of serotonin, while high frequency (70 Hz or greater) low intensity stimulation is employed to provoke endorphin release.

Current data from systematic reviews indicate that acupuncture is effective for dental pain and nausea, especially after surgery. Trials have shown no benefit of acupuncture in promoting smoking cessation or weight loss. Results are conflicting in the treatment of back pain, neck pain and tension headache. Contraindications to acupuncture include a tendency to bleeding; first trimester pregnancy (except when treating nausea) is also often considered a contraindication. The presence of a cardiac pacemaker precludes the use of electro-acupuncture, and indwelling needles must not be used in immuno-compromised patients at risk of infection. Bleeding, bruising and pain on needling are reported in 1-3% of cases. Serious side-effects are rare, but pneumothorax (collapsed lung) has been documented, as have fatalities. The use of sterile, disposable needles is clearly essential to prevent cross-infection.

Alexander technique

This technique is named after an Australian actor, Frederick Matthias Alexander. He developed the technique in the late 19th century in an attempt to prevent recurrent loss of his voice which he attributed to muscle tension in his head and neck. The most important underlying principle is that the relationship of the head, neck and spine is vital to enable the body to function at its best. Movement is considered to involve the least effort when the head leads and the spine follows. Teaching is given to correct posture and faulty movement patterns, usually to relieve back or neck pain or headaches. Repeated practice is thought to create new patterns or pathways of neuromuscular co-ordination, thereby improving posture, co-ordination and balance.

There is some evidence to support the view that the mind can initiate these changes, and it has been shown that the Alexander technique improves the efficiency of moving from a sitting to standing position. Studies have also shown that it can be effective in reducing back pain, and improve function in older people and patients with Parkinson's disease. The technique is safe and there are no known contraindications. It does however require considerable commitment on the part of the individual since 30 lessons lasting 45 to 60 minutes are recommended to learn the basic concepts, and some students embark on up to 100 lessons.

Aromatherapy

The use of plant oils to treat illness dates back to ancient Egypt, China and India. A French chemist, René Gattefosse, is credited in the 1930s with inspiring modern aromatherapy. On burning his hand in a perfume laboratory, he at once drenched it in lavender oil. The burn healed promptly without a scar, and he began to examine whether plant oils had curative properties. Essential plant oils can be administered by massage, added to bathwater, inhaled in hot water or diffused throughout a room. Scents from the oils activate the olfactory sense (smell) and trigger the limbic system, which regulates emotional responses, memory storage and retrieval. Smells can thus elicit memories and emotions which influence thoughts and feelings; the effects of plant oils can be relaxing or stimulating depending both on the chemistry of the particular oil and the individual's associations with a particular scent.

In 2000 a systematic review of randomised controlled trials of aromatherapy concluded that aromatherapy massage can produce a mild reduction in anxiety. Inconclusive results were obtained for the treatment of alopecia areata (a particular type of hair loss) and prevention of bronchitis; no benefit was found in treating perineal discomfort following childbirth.

Essential oils should not be taken internally or used undiluted on the skin. Some can cause photosensitivity and some are potentially carcinogenic. Allergic reactions are always a potential hazard. Essential oils can be expensive and are sometimes mixed with cheaper, synthetic oils.

Ayurvedic medicine

Ayurveda, the traditional medicine of India, dates back over 5,000 years. The Sanskrit word means 'knowledge of life' ('ayur' = life, 'veda' = knowledge) and encompasses a holistic approach to lifestyle incorporating medical, philosophical and religious beliefs. Health is thought to involve a balance of physical, mental, spiritual and environmental factors. Traditional Ayurvedic medicine teaches that life is sustained by a non-physical life energy called *prana* and that health requires a balanced flow of *prana*. Transcendental meditation is regarded as essential to reduce stress and induce altered states of consciousness. Other components of Ayurvedic medicine include *rasayanas* (herbal supplements), gemstones, purification procedures (leeches, sinus cleansing, purgatives, laxatives and enemas), chromotherapy (use of specific colours to induce healing), and religious ceremonies.

Few trials have compared herbal remedies with orthodox medication and there is currently limited evidence for the efficacy of Ayurvedic herbal treatments. As outlined previously, the safety of herbal remedies depends on purity and quality as well as the nature of the active ingredient.

Bach flower remedies

These were developed by Dr Edward Bach, a microbiologist working at the Royal London Homoeopathic Hospital in the early 1900s. Inspired by Hahnemann, the founder of homoeopathy, he attributed all illness to emotional imbalance. Based on his own experience while living in Wales he identified 38 flower remedies which he believed could treat most diseases by altering emotions. Bach alleged that the early rays of sunlight at dawn transferred the healing powers of the flowers into the dew accumulated on the petals. Later, in order to meet the demand for mass production, he suspended flowers in clear spring water and exposed them to direct sunlight, a practice still followed today. The remedies are supplied in concentrated solutions preserved in alcohol. Diluted, the infusions are then commonly taken internally in an attempt to balance physical and emotional disturbances; alternatively they can be applied to the skin.

Chemical analysis of Bach flower remedies reveals just water and alcohol. There are very few controlled clinical trials of their use; most are poorly designed and the results inconclusive. A randomised, placebo-controlled trial published in 2000 examined the value of the five flower *Rescue Remedy*, recommended as first aid treatment in emergencies, in reducing anxiety in 100 university students sitting examinations. There was no significant difference between *Rescue Remedy* and placebo. There are no known contraindications and little risk of adverse effects, although it should be noted they contain alcohol.

Biofeedback

B

Biofeedback relies on the principle that if an individual can be made aware of physiological responses in the body, he or she can learn to affect them. Traditional Eastern practices such as yoga and meditation have historically involved control of responses such as breathing and heart rate. In the 1960s Western researchers used electroencephalography (EEG) in volunteers to reproduce the brain's alpha waves. This was found to induce a state of deep relaxation and creative daydreaming, and to facilitate meditation. Simple attention is required, rather than conscious effort which may hinder the process, and the biofeedback device is used as an aid for a few sessions only until the individual has learnt to regulate their own responses. Any physiological response that can be monitored is suitable for biofeedback. Commonly used responses are electrical brain activity (EEG biofeedback), skin temperature (thermal), muscle tension (electromyography or EMG), blood pressure and respiratory rate.

Biofeedback is frequently used with other treatments such as cognitive therapy to assist in stress management and relaxation. There is clear evidence, especially using EEG, that individuals can alter physiological responses, although the precise mechanisms are unclear. Systematic reviews of clinical trials suggest that biofeedback is more effective than relaxation alone in managing tension headaches, migraines and children with attention deficit disorder.

Chiropractic medicine

The founder of chiropractic was a self-taught healer, Daniel David Palmer, a grocery store owner living in Iowa in the second half of the 19th century. Although spinal manipulation had been used for centuries beforehand, Palmer refined the technique with a series of manipulative procedures designed to restore health to muscles, nerves and organs considered to be out of alignment. He reasoned that disease was caused by misalignment, or subluxation, of the vertebral joints, causing excessive or inadequate pressure on spinal nerves. There has been controversy over the precise meaning of the term subluxation. Palmer and his son, Bartlett Joshua Palmer, are believed to have interpreted the term in a metaphysical sense to mean interference with the flow of energy through the body, while others seeking a rational explanation for chiropractic have interpreted subluxation as indicating displaced vertebrae which disrupt the flow of nerve impulses through the spine. Palmer termed the process chiropractic after the Greek *cheir* (hand) and *praxis* (action). While modern chiropractors use several manual therapeutic and diagnostic techniques, including massage and other joint-adjusting procedures, the most important is spinal manipulation, which applies high velocity low amplitude manual thrusts to spinal joints.

The principle that subluxation, metaphysical or physical, is the source of all illness has no scientific basis. Spinal mobilisation can however reduce muscle spasm and reduce the perception of pain. There is some evidence that spinal manipulation can be of benefit in treating acute low back pain, but not all the data support this conclusion. There is also some evidence to support its use in the treatment of non-migraine headaches.

Contraindications include advanced osteoporosis, bleeding disorders (including anticoagulant therapy), and malignant or inflammatory spinal disease. Serious side-effects are rare but include stroke. Up to half of patients report transient local discomfort after treatment.

Craniosacral therapy

C

This is a form of manipulation developed around 30 years ago by an osteopath, John Upledger, as a refinement of an older technique called cranial osteopathy. It is not however usually viewed as part of conventional osteopathic practice. It makes two assumptions. The first is that the bones of the cranium (skull) can be moved relative to one another. The second is that normal rhythmic impulses in the cerebrospinal fluid (CSF), which surrounds the brain and spinal cord, can be detected by palpation and may be restricted by the relative positions of the cranial bones. Craniosacral therapists aim to restore these impulses by moving the cranial bones through gentle manipulation.

Except in young babies, whose skulls have had to pass smoothly through the birth canal, only small movements are possible between cranial bones. There is no evidence that restrictions of these movements cause illness. In 1999 the Canadian Office of Health Technology Assessment published a review of the evidence for craniosacral therapy which concluded that there is insufficient evidence to support its use. Contraindications include any predisposition to, or actual, brain haemorrhage, and raised intracranial pressure. Although it has been suggested that young children respond especially well, caution seems prudent since their skull bones are still developing and in the process of fusing together.

Herbalism

Herbalism is defined as the therapeutic use of remedies containing only plant (or herb) material. Such preparations are taken internally or applied as creams. Examples include Ayurvedic and Chinese herbal remedies, kampo in Japan and phytomedicine or phytotherapy in modern Western societies.

As discussed in chapter four, plants have been used since the beginning of time for medicinal purposes. In the Genesis account of the domestic rivalry between Jacob's two wives, Rachel and Leah, reference is made to the ancient belief that the fruit of the mandrake plant has aphrodisiac properties (Genesis 30: 14-18). Modern Western herbalism, or phytomedicine, is incorporated into medical and pharmacy training in some European countries, for example Germany. Two points are worth noting. Firstly, in traditional herbal practice, patients with the same disease according to Western diagnostic criteria might receive very different herbal remedies. Secondly, in contrast to current phytotherapy practice, traditional herbal practice mainly makes use of complex mixtures of different herbs.

The rationale underlying all forms of herbalism is that the plant material used contains pharmacologically active ingredients which exert their effect at the cellular and molecular level to produce a biological response.

The clinical evidence for herbalism has to be evaluated depending on the individual preparation (as in modern phytotherapy) or according to the traditional practice. As outlined previously, there is evidence from clinical trials for the efficacy of some specific herbal remedies. These include saw palmetto for benign prostate gland enlargement, St John's Wort for mild to moderate depression, kava for anxiety and ginkgo biloba for certain circulatory problems. There is limited evidence for the efficacy of traditional Chinese and Ayurvedic herbal remedies.

Side-effects will vary according to the nature of the active ingredients. As discussed in chapter four, toxicity may also arise from contaminants if the quality of the product is substandard. Furthermore the potency of the active ingredient may vary between different preparations if not carefully regulated. Contraindications to herbal treatment must be considered individually depending on the constituents, but in most cases pregnancy and breast-feeding should be considered absolute contraindications.

Homoeopathy

H

This therapeutic method was formulated by Samuel Hahnemann (1755-1843) and was based on simple remedies (exercise, a nutritious diet and pure air) and two fundamental principles. The first of these is the so-called law of similars or 'like cures like' principle, which holds that symptoms are cured by drugs which produce in healthy persons the symptoms found in those who are ill. The second is the law of potentisation. This proposes that stepwise dilution, combined with vigorous shaking known as succussion, leads to increased potency. The process of dilution and succussion is claimed by some traditional homoeopathic practitioners to release a therapeutic 'immaterial and vital' force.

Homoeopathic remedies are labelled as so many 'x' or 'c'. For example, a 15x potency means that the original ingredient was diluted 15 times at a ratio of 1 in 10 (1 drop of the original solution mixed with 9 drops of water or alcohol). A 12c potency indicates that the original ingredient was diluted 12 times at a ratio of 1 in 100. Some remedies claimed to be effective are thus so dilute that they are likely to contain not a single molecule of the original active ingredient.

There is no evidence supporting the assumption that remedies containing no active ingredient can have clinical effects, although many possible explanations have been proposed. One idea which attracted popularity when published in the influential journal *Nature* in 1988 was that the original ingredient leaves an electromagnetic imprint on the surrounding water molecules. This idea, termed 'water memory', is not generally accepted, and the results of experiments described in the paper have not been reproduced. Some have likened the traditional explanation that succussion releases a spiritual, vital force, to the belief of Ayurvedic practitioners in *prana*.

The effectiveness of homoeopathic remedies has not been verified convincingly in clinical trials. Although adverse effects are likely to be few, in low dilutions some preparations can cause allergic reactions.

H Hypnotherapy

This can be defined as the induction of a trance-like state in order to facilitate relaxation and enhance suggestibility, with the ultimate goal of treating psychological or medical conditions and bringing about behavioural changes.

Hypnosis has been traced back to practice in ancient Egypt, but it is an Austrian physician Franz Anton Mesmer who is credited with its first therapeutic use in 1778. The term 'mesmerise' was derived from his practice. A Royal Commission which investigated his treatments based on magnetism concluded that his methods were entirely the result of imagination. It is James Braid, a British doctor, who is thought to have made hypnosis respectable among the medical community. The British and American Medical Associations subsequently legitimised hypnosis in the 1950s. Although hypnosis apparently results in an altered state of consciousness, a fundamental principle of practice is that the hypnotised individual remains in control, rather than the hypnotist or indeed others present.

Hypnosis is associated with a deep state of relaxation, the mechanism of which is not fully understood, and there is considerable controversy as to whether this genuinely represents an altered state of consciousness. Trust between the therapist and client is agreed to be vital. Some studies have suggested that hypnotherapy enhances the effects of psychotherapy in treating anxiety, insomnia, pain, increased blood pressure and obesity. A Cochrane review published in 1998 examined nine randomised controlled trials of smoking cessation and concluded that the technique was no more effective than placebo, and a further review of 59 studies published in 2000 supported these findings. A meta-analysis of 18 studies did however find in favour of hypnotherapy when used to treat pain. Benefit has also been reported in the treatment of some skin conditions, irritable bowel syndrome, and nausea and vomiting in cancer patients.

Contraindications include psychotic illness, personality disorders and epilepsy. It should not be used in children aged under five years. There are reports of information elicited under hypnosis being subject to confabulation (being made up), and also of false memory syndrome.

Iridology

I

Iridology uses examination of the eye to obtain information about the subject's health. It is based on the assumption that diseases of particular organs or regions are manifested by changes in specific locations in the iris. Neural connections between the iris and other body organs are proposed to explain the practice. Practitioners divide the iris into segments like those of a clock face. For example, it is thought that kidney disease is manifest in the right iris at the position of the hour hand at about 5.30, while thyroid disease would be manifest at about 2.30. The practice was developed in the 19th century by a Hungarian physician and gained popularity during the first part of the 20th century. Iridologists employ direct examination of the eye or study close-up photographs of the iris. In some countries travelling iridologists visit health food stores and conferences, take photographs of customers' eyes and then recommend herbal remedies or other products the practitioner considers appropriate either to prevent or treat disease.

It is well known that a wide number of medical conditions can affect the eyes generally. It is commonly the retina at the back of the eye which is affected, which is not visible on naked inspection or from ordinary close-up photographs. Common conditions affecting the retina include diabetes and high blood pressure. Less common conditions causing eye disease include certain inflammatory conditions and infections. There is however no evidence that the neural connections between body organs and the iris required to explain iridology exist, or that medical conditions affect any specific segment of the iris. A systematic review published in 2000 examined four controlled studies and concluded that iridology is neither valid nor useful.

Massage therapy

Massage describes a broad group of medical therapies that involve rubbing or moving the skin. There is evidence that massage is one of the oldest treatments known to mankind. Hippocrates is credited with saying that, 'The physician must be experienced in many things, but assuredly in rubbing'. A Swede, Per Henrik Ling, is credited with developing modern massage, also sometimes called Swedish massage, which involves manipulating the soft tissue of entire body areas using pressure and traction.

Massage fell out of favour in the early 20th century, doubtless partly because of the emerging availability of other, more effective, therapies; partly because it gained an association with sexual encounters (massage parlours had little to do with healthcare); and partly because physical touch came to be seen as inappropriate in a clinical context. Interest revived in the 1970s and in some European countries, such as Germany, massage is practised as part of orthodox medicine.

Massage employs various manual techniques, but touch is a fundamental component which enables the therapist to locate areas of muscle tension. Friction from the hands and mechanical pressure exerted on the skin and underlying structures enhance circulation and help to relieve muscular tension.

Systematic reviews have concluded that massage can be of benefit in treating constipation, low back pain, anxiety and fibromyalgia. A Cochrane review published in 1998 concluded that the evidence supporting its use to promote development in preterm and/or low birth weight infants was weak. Contraindications include deep vein thrombosis, burns, skin infections, eczema, open wounds, fractures and advanced osteoporosis. Caution should be exercised in patients suffering from cancer, those who have had a recent heart attack, and pregnant women. Patients embarking on massage therapy need to be comfortable with close physical contact. Adverse effects are extremely rare, but fractures and liver rupture have been reported. Allergic reactions can occur in response to the oils used in massage.

Naturopathy

N

Naturopathy aims to promote the body's own natural healing using a range of treatments such as clinical nutrition (which may include controlled fasting), acupuncture, counselling, herbal remedies, hydrotherapy, iridology and spinal manipulation. Naturopaths believe that life is more than a complex of biochemical processes, and that the body has an innate vitality which strives for health. The exact nature of this vitality varies according to the practitioner's views, some regarding it as merely a natural tendency towards health and others regarding it as a form of the life energy concept seen in Ayurvedic medicine. Health is considered not just to be the absence of disease, but rather a state which enables the individual to function well in a wide range of situations including those which are stressful. Seven principles have emerged which underpin this philosophy and are used in training naturopaths. The healing power of nature is emphasised, as is the need to identify and treat the cause of disease, to do no harm (by using safe and effective natural remedies), to treat the whole person, to educate the patient, to prevent disease through a healthy lifestyle and to establish health and wellness (defined as a positive emotional state despite the presence of disease) wherever possible.

The general principles of a healthy lifestyle, including a diet rich in fresh fruit and vegetables and regular physical exercise, have scientific validity and are not questioned by orthodox practitioners. The scientific validity of the different therapeutic methods employed by naturopaths depends on the methods used and the conditions they are employed to treat. Adverse effects and contraindications will differ according to each remedy employed.

Osteopathy

This manual therapy encompasses massage, mobilisation and spinal manipulation. It was Dr Andrew Taylor Still (1828-1917), a physician and Civil War surgeon in the Midwestern United States, who founded the practice. Osteopaths hold that the body has its own self-protecting and self-regulating mechanisms, that structure and function are closely related, and that problems in one organ affect other parts of the body. A perfect alignment of the musculoskeletal system is thought to eliminate obstructions in blood and lymphatic flow, and so optimise health. A range of manipulative techniques are employed which may include high velocity, low amplitude thrusts, craniosacral manoeuvres and counterstrain, in which tension is applied to restore normal musculoskeletal function.

There is no evidence supporting the view that perfect alignment of the musculoskeletal system is of overriding importance in maintaining overall health. Nevertheless there is evidence that osteopathy is effective in the treatment of low back pain, particularly when acute or subacute. Contraindications include osteoporosis, tumours, infections and a tendency to bleeding. Rare complications include spinal injury and stroke. It is generally considered that osteopathic techniques are gentler than those employed by chiropractic practitioners, and that the risk of spinal injury is thus less.

Reflexology

R

Reflexology is also sometimes known as 'zone therapy'. It uses manual pressure to specific areas of the feet, hands or ears which are thought to correspond to areas of the body. The aim is to prevent and treat physical conditions, and relieve stress.

The practice apparently dates back to ancient Egypt, where there is evidence of manual treatment of the feet, and such treatment was also seemingly part of Chinese culture. Zone therapy is recorded in North American Indian civilisation, and Dr William H Fitzgerald, an American ENT surgeon, derived the technique from American Indian practice. Although superficially resembling a foot massage, reflexology practitioners believe that the body is divided into ten vertical zones running from the feet to the head and down each arm, and that each zone is represented by a part of the foot including one toe. In the 1930s Eunice Ingham, a nurse and physical therapist, mapped out detailed reflex points on the feet. Examples include the idea that the tips of the three largest toes on both feet correspond to the brain, and that the left pelvis corresponds to the heel of the left foot. Proponents believe that application of pressure at the appropriate points breaks up granular accumulations of waste material (uric acid and calcium deposits) to allow free and balanced flow of energy and restoration of health.

There is no scientific evidence to support the idea that there are physiological connections between specific areas of the feet and certain organs or tissues. One blinded study has shown that reflexologists' diagnoses were no better than chance in identifying medical conditions, while another showed that diagnostic success was better than expected by chance alone but not clinically relevant. There are however no well-designed, large clinical studies, and foot massage may have general health benefits unrelated to the proposed mechanisms outlined above.

Contraindications include conditions such as gout, foot ulcers or impaired circulation in the lower limbs; caution is advised if patients are suffering from bone or joint disease in the feet. Foot tenderness and allergy to oils, if used, are potential side-effects.

Reiki

The term Reiki is derived from the Japanese *rei*, which means universal, and *ki*, which means vital force. *Ki* is the Japanese term for *prana*, or *chi*, the universal life energy in Ayurvedic and Chinese traditions. It is also sometimes referred to as spiritual healing, therapeutic touch or faith healing. Some claim that Reiki was practised by Buddha and in 1st century Rome. Some have also claimed that Reiki was practised by Jesus Christ; closer examination (see below under Spiritual healing) shows these claims are not substantiated by biblical evidence.

Modern Reiki was developed by a Zen Buddhist monk, Mikao Usui, after his experiences during a three week fast on Mount Koriyama in Japan in the mid 1800s. All Reiki practices hold that a divine, healing life energy pervades each person and that illness arises when energy flow through the person is blocked. The Reiki practitioner acts as a channel directing the Reiki energy to flow freely towards the patient. Reiki training involves the practitioner learning to be open to the energy; the energy itself is thought to know what each patient needs for healing. Training involves Reiki Masters, who call upon the help of spirit guides. Training is in several stages and practitioners are described as being either first or second degree, or third degree Masters. Until recently Reiki was only performed in secret ceremonies. Therapeutic sessions usually involve touch from the therapist; however second and third degree practitioners claim to be able to send energy over long distances and are thus not required physically to be present for healing to occur.

There is no scientific evidence to support the existence of an independent, healing energy and there are no good quality clinical trials validating the use of Reiki. There are no formal contraindications to Reiki. Christians, who are instructed not to embark on communication with spirits and spirit guides, should clearly not pursue it.

Relaxation therapy

R

Relaxation therapy employs techniques which elicit a so-called 'relaxation response' from the autonomic nervous system. The commonest technique is called progressive muscle relaxation, which was developed in 1930 by an American physician, Dr Edmund Jacobson. This proposes that tension in any part of the body is impossible if the muscles are completely relaxed. Tension in involuntary muscles and organs is thought to be reduced if the associated skeletal, or voluntary, muscles are relaxed. Voluntary muscle relaxation is learnt by first distinguishing between muscle tension and relaxation; later the patient learns to relax the muscles without having to tense them first.

Progressive muscle relaxation has been shown to improve blood supply to muscles, reduce oxygen consumption and heart rate, and diminish muscle activity associated with breathing. Other techniques have been shown to diffuse muscle tension.

There is considerable evidence to suggest that relaxation techniques are useful in treating anxiety, although they do not appear to be as effective as psychotherapy. Randomised controlled trials have shown benefit in agoraphobia (fear of open spaces) and those suffering from panic attacks. Systematic reviews of its use in acute and chronic pain are less convincing. Some studies suggest potential for relaxation therapy in the treatment of depression, insomnia and menopausal symptoms, although the effects appear to be short-lived.

Contraindications include psychosis; depressed mood can be worsened by some relaxation techniques.

S Shiatsu

Shiatsu is a Japanese form of massage strongly influenced by traditional Chinese medicine. Developed from acupressure, it employs finger pressure, or *shiatsu*, on hundreds of surface points of the body. It was originally developed to detect and treat problems with the flow of life energy, or *ki*.

Shiatsu is scientifically unproven, although the acupressure and massage components themselves may be helpful in relieving stress, tension and pain. Shiatsu practised with the hands is generally safe from a physical standpoint, but bruising may occur when practitioners use their elbows or feet to deliver the therapy. As for Reiki, there are no formal contraindications, but patients should be aware that some Shiatsu practitioners may call on spiritual forces to assist in healing.

Spiritual healing

S

Spiritual healing is a broad umbrella term encompassing a range of practices by individuals and practitioners with very different faith systems. Hence it is often grouped together with other practices such as Reiki, therapeutic touch, psychic healing and paranormal healing. In this non-specific sense it is defined as a direct interaction between two individuals, one who is the healer and one who is sick, with the intention of improving or curing illness. Energy of one kind or another is believed to be transferred to the patient via the healer; emotional problems or chronic pain are often addressed in this context.

Spiritual healing has been traced back to the New Testament (1 Corinthians 12:9), where it is cited as a divine gift. The story of Jesus healing the woman with a haemorrhage of 12 years' duration illustrates the problem many face when trying to distinguish between the approaches employed. When the woman in the busy crowd touched the edge of Jesus' coat and was immediately healed, he recognised at once that 'power has gone out from me' (Luke 8:46). Superficially this bears similarities to Reiki (see above), but it is clearly important to discern where the healing is thought to come from. In the Bible it is God alone, his power mediated through Jesus Christ and the Holy Spirit, who is the source of all healing. Communication with spirit guides, as in Reiki, is in clear opposition to Christian teaching and would be regarded as part of occult practice denounced in the Old Testament (see for example Leviticus 19:26).

A systematic review of 23 randomised controlled trials of spiritual healing involving nearly 3,000 patients and published in 2000 could not draw any firm conclusions as to its efficacy. Studies of prayer for physical and psychological conditions are also inconclusive. Christians should not be surprised that such 'prayer research' shows no clear benefits, since some of the prayer employed was not Christian in origin. Furthermore, even studies of Christian prayer are based on the assumption that only humans impact the results, and that if prayer works, what is prayed for will come about. This approach thus presupposes that prayer is impersonal. In contrast, Biblical prayer is based on an inherently personal encounter with a loving God and should never become merely mechanical. Christian theologians throughout history have acknowledged the reality and the pain of the mystery of unanswered prayer, as illustrated by Paul's unanswered prayer for God to remove a 'thorn in my flesh' (2 Corinthians 12:7).

T

Tai Chi

This is a system of gentle movements and graceful postures, based on ancient Chinese philosophy and martial arts and used to improve physical and psychological well-being. Tai Chi, or Tai Chi Chuan, literally means 'supreme ultimate power'. Inspired by Confucian and Buddhist thinking, it is based on the principle of opposing life forces, yin (the female, receptive principle) and yang (the male, creative principle). Practising outdoors, especially early in the morning, is favoured because it is thought to facilitate the flow of universal *chi* in the earth through the feet to replenish the individual's own *chi*. The degree to which the spiritual basis is emphasised will depend on the practitioner.

There is limited evidence from well-designed clinical trials. Nevertheless the scientific evidence does suggest that Tai Chi can help maintain balance and strength, reduce risk of falls and improve cardio-respiratory function in elderly individuals, and lessen depression and anxiety. Contraindications include severe osteoporosis, acute back pain, knee problems, sprains and fractures. Adverse effects are rare but can include muscle soreness, pulled ligaments and ankle sprains.

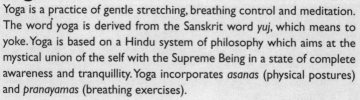

Yoga

Yoga is a practice of gentle stretching, breathing control and meditation. The word yoga is derived from the Sanskrit word *yuj*, which means to yoke. Yoga is based on a Hindu system of philosophy which aims at the mystical union of the self with the Supreme Being in a state of complete awareness and tranquillity. Yoga incorporates *asanas* (physical postures) and *pranayamas* (breathing exercises).

Regular yoga practice induces a state of deep relaxation which confers at least transient benefit. A small number of controlled studies suggest it may be of benefit in reducing high blood pressure and reducing stiffness in patients with osteoarthritis. There are no absolute contraindications but certain postures are contraindicated in pregnancy. Yoga is not recommended for those with a history of psychosis or personality disorder. Potential side effects include drowsiness and muscular or ligamentous strain. Although the practice of yoga does not oblige students to hold specific spiritual beliefs or follow religious observances, enthusiastic adherents are likely to observe Eastern spiritual practices.

Further reading

1. Ernst E (Ed). *The Desktop guide to Complementary and Alternative Medicine: an evidence-based approach.* UK: Mosby, 2001
2. Jonas W, Levin J. *Essentials of Complementary and Alternative Medicine.* USA: Lippincott Williams & Wilkins, 1999
3. O'Mathuna D, Larimore W. *Alternative Medicine: The Christian Handbook.* USA: Zondervan, 2001

8

Assessing CAM therapies

In chapter six I suggested some ways in which we could seek to evaluate new therapies being offered. I will now present some fictional case histories or scenarios, designed to illustrate how one might attempt to apply some specific questions to CAM therapies. The aim of this exercise is to help the reader to develop his or her own ideas about how to assess CAM treatments. The scenarios (in the shaded boxes) can be used by the reader alone, or you might want to use them in a small group as a starting point for discussion about CAM. I have tried to make them as close to real life situations as possible; and I hope that medical and non-medical readers alike will find them relevant and of interest. They can be varied for use in different settings or as an aid to finding out the facts about a particular therapy.

A few words of caution are needed here. Firstly, assumptions made in this book about the current state of scientific evidence for any one CAM therapy will soon be outdated. Thus, what is thought to be true today may not be true in tomorrow's world. Obviously this limitation does not apply to unchanging truths, such as the nature of God or evil, but it does mean that this model does not represent a set of unchanging rules.

Secondly, as I concluded in chapter six, God gives individuals free choice. There are undoubtedly principles which God does not intend us to violate. I mentioned some of these briefly in the Introduction. We are not to murder or to steal. There is absolute truth. However, every individual is unique, with different personal circumstances and upbringing. There are also some questions to which we will never know the full answer in this life. On such controversial matters Paul wrote, '"Everything is permissible" – but not everything is beneficial. "Everything is permissible" – but not everything is constructive...So whether you eat or drink or whatever you do, do it all for the glory of God' (1 Corinthians 10:23, 31).

Scenario 1

You have a friend who has suffered from low back pain for 18 months. Treatment from his general practitioner with simple painkillers has produced little benefit and he is considering consulting an osteopath. He knows you are reading a book on CAM therapies and he asks you for your advice.

Questions for thought and/or discussion:

What else would you want to know?
What would be your advice?

This scenario illustrates one of the most important and common potential pitfalls presented by CAM, which I have not yet addressed. On the face of it the answer to your friend's question seems fairly straightforward. You have been reading about osteopathy and you know there is evidence that it can be safe and effective in the treatment of low back pain. You also happen to know of a local osteopath who works in the nearby GP surgery and who has also been recommended by one of your friends on the basis of their own experience.

However, before you can go ahead and recommend osteopathy, you must know more about his back pain. Although statistically unlikely, your friend could have an undiagnosed cancer. In that case recourse to osteopathy would cause him harm by delaying access to conventional diagnosis and treatment. Your advice to him must be that he should go back to his general practitioner and ask whether he or she thinks osteopathy might be helpful or at the very least safe, or if not, whether further tests are required first to establish the cause of his back pain.

Scenario 2

Your teenage daughter has asthma which has been quite troublesome over the past few years and on one occasion necessitated an overnight stay in hospital. Over breakfast one Saturday morning she informs you she has taken up a yoga class with her friends and feels very much better. She has already halved the dose of her brown (steroid) inhaler of her own accord and plans to stop it altogether next month.

Questions for thought and/or discussion:

What else would you like to know?
What would be your advice?

Leaving aside the consideration of whether your daughter is likely to take your advice, there are at least three issues here. The first is whether you are comfortable with your daughter attending a yoga class. The second is whether yoga has any proven benefit in treating asthma. The third is whether it is sensible for her to stop her asthma medication without getting medical advice first.

Assuming you don't know very much about yoga, and particularly its use in asthma, how should you proceed? You may consult this book, or one of the books listed at the end of chapter 7, but you may also want to get information from the internet. How can you ensure that you obtain high quality information about CAM therapies from the internet? In Box 1 at the end of this chapter I have outlined some general tips for searching for high quality healthcare information on the internet.

Let us imagine you find a review of three studies by a respected author in the field. One of these examined over 100 subjects; of these, those who continued to practise yoga regularly over four years showed a significant reduction in asthma medication use and improved peak flow readings compared with the control group. However, there was a high drop out rate. Two further studies failed to show any improvement in breathing measurements, although yoga did have a favourable effect on mood. The review concludes that the benefits of yoga in asthma are not clearly established, and that it should not be used alone to treat asthma. Nevertheless yoga appears to have some benefits for those are motivated to persevere with it long-term.

It is also important to ask whether it is the principle, or the method which is effective (see Box 2). In the case of yoga it is not necessarily the principle of meditation (a specifically spiritual activity) which is effective, but the method of the technique. Any equally relaxing activity should produce the same physiological benefits.

Regardless of the medical evidence, whether you are comfortable with your daughter attending a yoga class will depend on your interpretation of yoga as taught in the West, and on the world view of the teacher. Many believe that the practice of yoga in the West does not oblige students to hold specific spiritual beliefs or follow religious observances. Nevertheless, as mentioned in chapter seven, enthusiastic proponents are likely to observe Eastern spiritual practices.

Finally, there is the important question of your daughter abandoning her orthodox medicine in favour of a much more pleasant, sociable activity. Asthma, although often mild, can be under-recognised and under-treated even by doctors, and there is no doubt that it can be life-threatening. Stopping conventional treatment is another potential hazard of taking up CAM without sufficient knowledge or medical advice, and could be dangerous.

You may conclude from the above that there is insufficient evidence that your daughter will benefit from yoga, and that you are unhappy about its spiritual connotations. Even if she insists on continuing to attend the class, she should certainly be advised not to stop her treatment and to consult her own general practitioner who can explain the risks to her of stopping treatment.

Scenario 3

You visit your parents. Your mother, who is aged 72 and leads an active life, has just been diagnosed with osteoarthritis. She asks you whether you would recommend glucosamine and chondroitin supplements. She has read an article about them in a free magazine from the local health food store and is very keen to give them a try.

Question for thought and/or discussion:
What would be your advice?

Your reading leads you to conclude that glucosamine and chondroitin are probably better than placebo in the treatment of osteoarthritis. There are no spiritual implications, and you feel able to recommend that she goes ahead.

However, you do tell her that the benefit is probably modest, that she should buy a product sold by a reputable health store, and that she will need to match the doses used in clinical trials, such as 1.5 g of glucosamine and 800-1,200mg of chondroitin daily. You also warn her that such products can be expensive (typically £20-£30 a month) and she may want to consider a three month trial, at the end of which she may want to review how helpful she thinks it has been.

It would also be sensible for her to let her general practitioner know she is taking it.

Scenario 4

During the time you spend visiting your parents, your mother also confides that she has bought some saw palmetto for your father, because of his 'prostate problems'.

Questions for thought and/or discussion:

What else would you want to know?

What would be your advice?

As in Scenario 1, the potential risk here is that your father's health problem is misdiagnosed, or that the diagnosis is delayed, if he has recourse to CAM therapies without first obtaining medical advice. Although benign prostate disease is common in older men, so is prostate cancer, and the initial symptoms can be similar. It is therefore vital that he sees his general practitioner for a check-up, if he has not done so recently, to ascertain that he does not have prostate cancer. Saw palmetto will be of no benefit to him if he did, and could cause harm by delaying access to effective orthodox treatments.

Assuming your father does indeed have benign prostate disease, you will want to know whether there is any evidence that saw palmetto could help relieve some or all of the symptoms, and whether it is safe.

Saw palmetto is a dwarf palm native to the coast region of southern states in the USA. In traditional American medicine it was used to treat bladder or urethral irritations, and between 1906 and 1950 the US Pharmacopeia and National Formulary included a reference to saw palmetto tea as a remedy for urogenital ailments. In the 21st century it remains popular, especially in Germany, for treating the symptoms of benign prostate enlargement.

A systematic review published in 1998 assessed 18 randomised controlled trials of saw palmetto in benign prostate disease, and concluded that it significantly improves symptoms and urinary flow compared with placebo. When compared with the drug usually prescribed by NHS doctors, finasteride, saw palmetto also had fewer side-effects. Several further studies appear to confirm these findings, although there are no long-term data available. Side-effects include diarrhoea or constipation, and reduced libido.

You may therefore conclude that saw palmetto is an attractive option for your father, and decide to recommend it to him. You make it clear that he needs to purchase it from a reputable supplier; the usual dose is 320mg daily in divided doses.

He should let his general practitioner know if he follows your suggestion.

Scenario 5

You attend a family reunion. Your cousin, who has just reached the menopause, knows you are interested in CAM therapies and asks what your views are on 'over-the-counter herbal remedies' for her troublesome symptoms.

Question for thought and/or discussion:
What will you say to her?

A number of CAM approaches have been proposed. Reviews show that the most popular are dietary nutritional supplements, spiritual approaches, physical exercise, herbal medicines and homoeopathy. None of these is convincingly effective, especially when their effects are compared with those of the orthodox approach, that of hormone replacement therapy. Furthermore, many have potential side-effects which must be taken into account before embarking on a course of treatment. The most promising herbal remedies at present are black cohosh, kava and soy supplements; relaxation techniques also appear to be beneficial.

You could probably therefore suggest to your cousin that she considers trying black cohosh, kava and soy supplements. She would be wise to do some reading first so she is aware of the side-effects, and only buy them from a reputable supplier to ensure quality.

It would also be prudent for her to let her doctor know she is taking them, particularly if she is taking other medication.

Scenario 6

A friend/colleague wants to set up an acupuncture service and consults you for your views.

Question for thought and/or discussion:

What issues will you want to discuss? You can adapt this to your own situation, whether you are a member of the public with an interest in CAM, or a healthcare professional based in primary or secondary care.

Assuming you don't have reason to believe that the service is untenable, there is a wide range of issues which can be considered. If you are a member of the public you will have views on the facilities which should be available, and on accessibility (for example whether evening and weekend appointments should be offered). You will doubtless have concerns shared by healthcare professionals, such as regulation and safety.

In the community, successful acupuncture services have been set up alongside primary care practices, sometimes offered with a range of other CAM therapies such as osteopathy. An example is the Glastonbury Integrated Healthcare Centre in Somerset, where savings made on referrals to secondary care have been used to help fund the CAM service. The clear advantages here are that the service can be monitored or even regulated by the GP surgery, and general practitioners can refer to the service when considered appropriate. The surgery will have the final decision over who is employed to offer the service, and there will be a framework for ensuring safety requirements, such as use of disposable needles and adequate training.

In secondary care, the constraints will be greater, but there will be a similar emphasis on employing a practitioner with appropriate qualifications. Very often this will be an orthodox anaesthetist trained in acupuncture. Advertising of the service will be limited and referrals likely to come from healthcare professionals within the organisation.

It becomes clear, therefore, that the prime considerations are those of ensuring patient safety. Where there is some evidence to support the use of a particular CAM therapy, such as acupuncture and osteopathy, an association with an existing NHS practice has the advantage that the service can be monitored or regulated by the NHS body. This should prevent practitioners who are unsuitably qualified from setting up and running the service. Where there is little or no evidence to support the practice, association with NHS organisations has the disadvantage that it confers respectability on a therapy with dubious credentials. This should be taken into account in all such planning.

Conclusions

With some background information, assuming balanced and intelligent sources, it is now possible to find out a reasonable amount about any one particular CAM therapy and develop informed views about whether one wishes to adopt this approach.

As I outlined in chapter six, the key issues Christians will want to consider will not only be the quality of the scientific evidence supporting the practice, but also the therapist's world-view and their motives.

Box 1
Tips for searching the internet for healthcare information

Use a reputable search engine (such as Google or its environmentally friendly cousin Blackle)

Use reputable websites, such as those provided by national bodies providing patient and consumer information (see Appendix)

Avoid websites which clearly are largely based on anecdotal evidence or personal experience, or which use inflammatory, emotional and/or defamatory language

If you want to deepen your search, use professional websites which use specific criteria for inclusion of material, for instance the medical journal search engine Pubmed

In order to avoid being overwhelmed with evidence from dozens or hundreds of studies, limit your preliminary searches to reviews

Consider searching specifically for reviews of articles by a reputable author whom you know is respected in the field. An example in the UK is Professor Edzard Ernst from Exeter

If you are unsure how to get the best out of an internet search engine or literature searching site, follow the advice given on the site, buy a book on the subject, or consult your local library

---

Box 2

Questions to ask when assessing a CAM therapy

Do the claims made for this therapy fit the facts?

Is there a rational scientific basis for the therapy?

Is the methodology or the principle the effective element?

What is the therapist's world-view?

Does the therapy involve the occult?

Box 3

Summary of possible side effects when using CAM

Recourse to CAM may delay accurate diagnosis

Recourse to CAM may give the patient false confidence and lead them to reduce or stop prescription medicines

The ingredients in herbal remedies may be unknown, toxic, or there may be contamination

The ingredients in herbal remedies may interact with prescribed medicines

CAM usually entails financial costs which must be weighed against the possible benefits

There may be spiritual hazards if the therapy is based on spiritual principles which conflict with a Christian worldview

Appendix:
Useful healthcare websites providing information on CAM

1. General sites

These sites all cover a wide range of healthcare related issues. They can help provide information on organisations offering and regulating CAM, the scientific background for a particular CAM therapy, and the evidence for its safety and efficacy. However, they do not usually address spiritual aspects, so the reader who is concerned about these may need to consult other sources to find information on any spiritual principles involved.

Bandolier
www.jr2.ox.ac.uk/bandolier/
This site features carefully researched articles and reviews on a variety of subjects, not just CAM, presented in a format accessible to the public as well as healthcare professionals. It also contains guidance about how to appraise research articles. The Healthy Living Zone in particular includes information on CAM.

BMC Complementary and Alternative Medicine
www.biomedcentral.com/bmccomplementalternmed/
This site features an open access journal publishing original peer-reviewed research articles on complementary and alternative healthcare interventions.

CAM Specialist Library
www.library.nhs.uk/cam/
As its title suggests, this site is devoted specifically to research on CAM. It is provided by the NHS National Library for Health.

Cochrane Collaboration
www.cochrane.org/
This site provides up-to-date evidence and reviews on a wide variety of healthcare topics. It is largely intended for use by healthcare professionals, but it includes clearly written 'plain language summaries' aimed at the public.

Complementary Medicine Unit, Exeter University
www.pms.ac.uk/compmed/
This department publishes a quarterly review journal, FACT (*Focus on Alternative and Complementary Therapies*), whose stated aims are to present the evidence on CAM in an analytical and impartial manner. The journal is edited by Professor Ernst and can be accessed directly at **www.ex.ac.uk/FACT**. Sample summaries are available online or there is the option to subscribe regularly.

Journal of Alternative and Complementary Medicine
www.liebertpub.com
This is the site for Mary Ann Liebert, Inc, which publishes journals in a variety of fields including biomedical research. This includes the *Journal of Alternative and Complementary Medicine*.

Medicines and Healthcare Products Regulatory Agency (MHRA)
www.mhra.gov.uk
This site is mainly aimed at healthcare professionals but also has articles for the public, including a particularly useful consumer guide to using herbal medicines.

Pub Med
www.ncbi.nlm.nih.gov/sites/entrez
This site is provided by the US National Library of Medicine and contains millions of articles published in high quality peer-reviewed scientific journals in a broad range of biomedical fields. Intended for professionals, it is nevertheless open access and thus available to the public. It has links to a tutorial on searching the database.

2. Disease specific sites

These are websites run by professional organisations focusing on one particular disease or organ, for example the kidneys or the lungs. Sponsored by charities and largely aimed at the public and patients, they provide varying amounts of information on CAM in a disease specific setting. However, because their main focus is on orthodox therapies, it is usually necessary to search the site for a specific term.

Arthritis Research Campaign
www.arc.org.uk

British Lung Foundation
www.lunguk.org

Cancerbackup
www.cancerbackup.org.uk/Home
Cancerbackup is Europe's leading cancer information charity. The site contains over 4,500 pages of up-to-date information on cancer for patients and their families.

Cancer Research UK
www.cancerresearchuk.org/

Complementary Therapies in Clinical Practice
www.sciencedirect.com/science/journal/17443881
This journal publishes articles on CAM research. Abstracts are available on the site; access to full articles requires a subscription.

Diabetes UK
www.diabetes.org.uk/

Parkinson's Disease
www.parkinson.org.uk/

Verity
www.verity-pcos.org.uk
This site contains information for patients with polycystic ovary syndrome (PCOS). Verity publishes an information pack purchased online or offered free with membership. The pack includes information on CAM therapies for PCOS.

Index